the little book of
self-care
for
mums-to-be

Beccy Hands and
Alexis Stickland

Illustrations by Kay Train

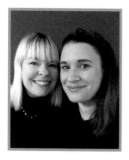

Beccy Hands is a doula and remedial massage therapist specialising in pre- and postnatal wellbeing, who has been supporting women since 2003.

Alexis Stickland is a midwife, antenatal teacher and mother of three children who has been supporting women and their families since 2004.

Together they founded The Mother Box in 2017, a company that supports expectant and new mums with essential advice and nurturing wellbeing gift boxes.

Kay Train is a freelance illustrator whose work has appeared in bestselling books and national publications. www.kaytrain.com @kaytrainillustrator

10 9 8 7 6 5 4 3 2

Vermilion, an imprint of Ebury Publishing,
20 Vauxhall Bridge Road,
London, SW1V 2SA

Vermilion is part of the Penguin Random House group of companies whose addresses can be found at global.penguinrandomhouse.com

 Penguin Random House UK

www.penguin.co.uk

First published by Vermilion in 2020

A CIP catalogue record for this book is available from the British Library

Commissioning Editor: Samantha Jackson
Project Editor: Laura Herring
Designer: Laura Liggins and Nikki Dupin at Studio nic&lou
Illustrator: Kay Train

ISBN 9781785042959

Printed and bound in Italy

Penguin Random House is committed to a sustainable future for our business, our readers and our planet. This book is made from Forest Stewardship Council® certified paper.

 MIX
Paper from responsible sources
FSC® C018179
www.fsc.org

The information in this book has been compiled by way of general guidance in relation to the specific subjects addressed. It is not a substitute and not to be relied on for medical, healthcare, pharmaceutical or other professional advice on specific circumstances and in specific locations. Please consult your GP before changing, stopping or starting any medical treatment. So far as the authors are aware the information given is correct and up to date as at March 2020. Practice, laws and regulations all change, and the reader should obtain up to date professional advice on any such issues. The authors and publishers disclaim, as far as the law allows, any liability arising directly or indirectly from the use, or misuse, of the information contained in this book.

Contents:

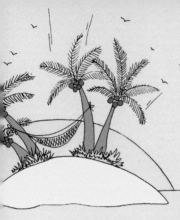

adventure awaits

Congratulations, you are about to embark on one of the most significant adventures of your life. Pregnancy really is amazing, magical and exciting. The fact that you can grow an actual human being, birth and then care for them still blows our minds all these years later. Pregnancy is a gift and we are well aware that for some, there may have been an epic journey to get to this point, making it an even more wondrous and emotional experience.

Having said that, we also know it can be challenging, leaving you open to vulnerability, and feeling like you're on your knees with exhaustion at times. It's a rollercoaster and all of your feelings are completely valid. From morning sickness (totally misbranded, as it can often last all day) and hormonal headaches to swollen feet and ankles, and varicose veins in places you'd rather not have them, we've seen it all and we have a secret to share: you don't have to put up with heartburn, you can do something for pelvic pain, and you can help those pesky piles go away quicker.

We have seen what a difference it makes when a woman truly cares for herself, supports her incredible body as it changes, allows herself time to rest, and finds support when she needs it. But to really be able to do this for ourselves, first we have to understand why things are happening, and what we can do about it. After all, we don't know until we know, right? We've filled this book with as many little tips and tricks as we could fit in it, to give you some easy and inexpensive ideas for how best to support your body through the trimesters as it adapts to cater for your little bean's every need. Often the best remedies are actually in our kitchen cupboards and we want to show you how you can make use of them throughout your pregnancy.

Having had the absolute honour of training abroad, in cultures where women are truly nurtured and celebrated during pregnancy and birth (and beyond), and seeing what a wonderful impact that has on their physical and mental wellbeing, we wanted to create a book that brought a little bit of this knowledge to your bedside table.

Don't forget that each pregnancy is unique, so even if this isn't your first baby, this book will still be as valuable to you as it will be to a first-time mum. We want to support you with any worry or symptom that you might be experiencing, and have suggested simple and effective ways that you can care for yourself and have confidence in supporting your changing body.

We know how busy life can be, so we have kept the sections short and snappy so you can dip in and out of them easily. So, whatever is bothering you during these next nine months, we hope you will find a little tip, trick or fist bump in here to make you feel held, cared for and truly celebrated for the queen that you are!

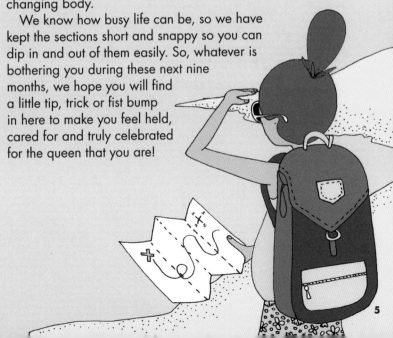

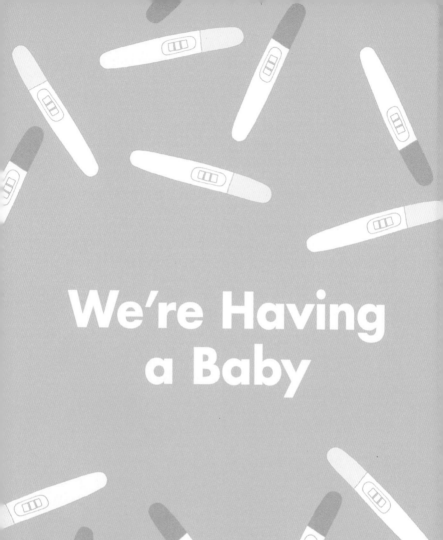

We're Having a Baby

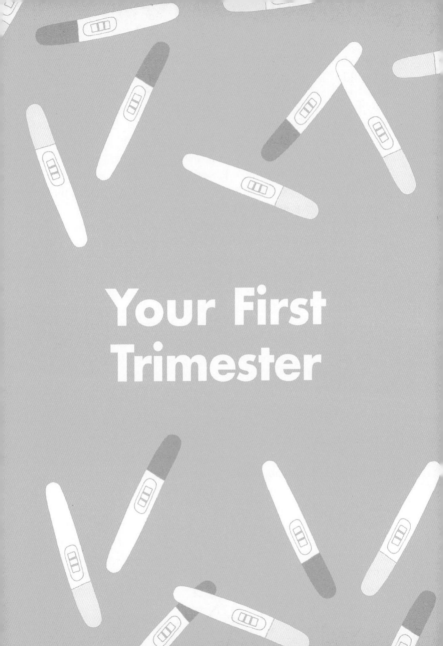

Your First Trimester

Huge congratulations on the exciting news that you are growing your very own tiny human! Even after all these years of working with pregnant women, the discovery that there is a new baby on the way remains as magical as ever.

The first twelve weeks of your pregnancy is such an incredible period of mentally processing your big news and adapting to changes in both your mind and body. You are truly amazing and right now the growth and development of your tiny baby (or babies) is rapid! It's fascinating to think that even though your little one may only be the size of a lime by the end of the first trimester, the lion's share of development will have already taken place and you may already notice some changes starting to happen.

With all of this going on, it is hardly surprising you may feel physically drained, nauseous and emotional during these early weeks. Taking time and making a conscious effort to care for yourself is not self-indulgent, it's a necessity, and it will benefit you hugely, not only now but also in the long run.

Like many mums-to-be, you may have chosen to keep the news to yourself for now, which means there are probably very few people in the know to offer guidance or an extra dose of TLC to carry you through. That's where we come in! We don't want you to feel alone now or at any point during your pregnancy, so turn to these pages for a quick pick-me-up, some reassurance and practical ideas to help keep you as comfortable as possible during your first trimester.

You may keep looking at your positive pregnancy test in disbelief and wondering whether this is a normal reaction?! Worry not! Many expectant parents have said that it took a significant time for them to digest the enormity of their newly confirmed pregnancy.

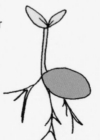

So don't be surprised if you feel a little shocked and bewildered to begin with, even if this was a long time in the planning. At this early stage, the reality that those two blue lines are going to transform over the next nine months into a tiny scrummy bundle of baby is so abstract that it's completely understandable if your brain bubbles are taking their time processing the news. Pregnancy, birth and motherhood are likely to be on your mind a lot right now and it can feel daunting that so much of this journey is still unknown. However, there is also so much to experience and look forward to as you begin your motherhood adventure, so let's dive in!

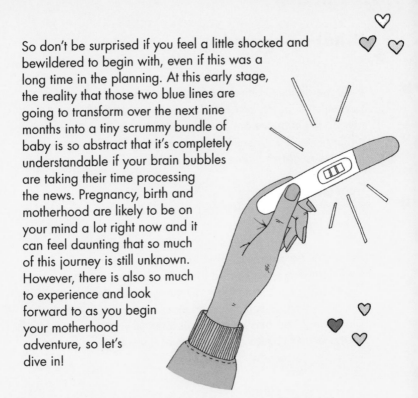

TO TELL OR NOT TO TELL?
How and when you share your news with friends, family and colleagues is a very personal decision. Many women mention that they feel a little superstitious and would rather share their news once they have had their first scan at twelve weeks. Some women choose to tell a select few special people, while others are happy to discuss their pregnancy openly from the day they find out. Whatever you decide to do, it might be helpful to consider how you are feeling physically and mentally and whether it would be beneficial to have some VIPs to lean on for support as you navigate your way through the peaks and pits of your first trimester.

What's happening?

It can be difficult in these early days to understand exactly how much is going on behind the scenes, because from the outside the changes are so subtle. Inside, however, is a totally different story. Your entire body is working like a pregnancy machine to get you through this first trimester.

Hormones
Some of the most significant changes in the first trimester are caused by the huge surge of pregnancy hormones, namely oestrogen and progesterone, travelling through your body. This rapid increase in oestrogen is responsible for many women feeling sickness and fatigue in those early weeks. The good news is that higher progesterone levels are also thought to lead to some women experiencing a pregnancy 'glow', thick hair and healthy nails later down the line. Shifting hormones may cause other symptoms, including:

- frequent weeing
- tender boobs: ease the discomfort by wearing a well-fitting, comfy bra — avoid underwired bras as they can put too much pressure on the sensitive tissue
- sluggish digestion
- increased watery vaginal discharge
- hormonal headaches
- sleep disturbances
- an intense sense of taste and smell
- a metallic taste in the mouth
- spotty, sallow skin

Now you can see why it's completely normal for you to also experience mood changes and to find yourself feeling more emotional than usual. Some women find tolerating these symptoms a bit easier once they understand the important and positive reasons behind these acute hormonal changes:

OESTROGEN
· Increases the essential blood circulation and blood flow to your womb
· Supports the growth and maintenance of your uterine lining
· Supports your developing babe
· Helps to transfer nutrients to your little one

PROGESTERONE
· Aids the loosening of ligaments and joints
· Transforms internal structures and enables them to increase in size, such as the uterus growing from the size of a small pear to the size of a large watermelon
· Helps prevent uterine contractions until labour
· Prevents established lactation until birth

While you are travelling through your first trimester, rapid amounts of growth and development are also happening to your baby. Your body is working super-hard to create and maintain a supportive, nurturing environment for your little one, with very little conscious effort from you. In a few short months, your foetus will have gone from a cell, barely detectable, to being recognisable on a scan as a baby. Their brain and spinal cord have been developing and expanding, their heart has gone from nothing to a flutter to a beat, their sex organs are present and their little legs, toes, fingers and arms have taken form. It's mind-blowing when you think about it.

REMEMBER: every woman and every pregnancy is different. How pronounced your pregnancy symptoms feel — whether you experience all of the symptoms above or none — and how you adjust to the physical and mental changes will be as unique as you.

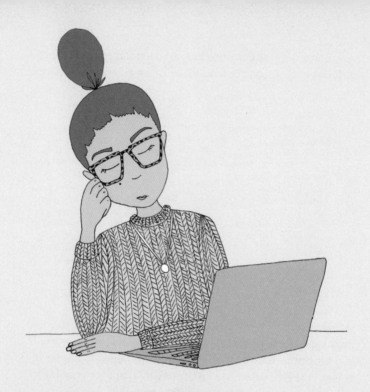

Tiredness Like No Other

Why do I feel so bone-tired? Well first, let's remember what's happening here: apart from the crazy hormones and the fact you are slowly growing a real-life actual human being, you are also having to use all of your energy reserves to create a life-support machine for that little baby, which entails making a whole other organ from scratch – this is your placenta!

This is why it really is important to listen to your body and allow yourself to rest as much as you can in the first trimester. Thankfully, the tiredness should ease up by the second trimester, when your placenta has fully formed and your hormones have settled a little. Although do be prepared that this tiredness may creep back again around the third trimester, as your baby grows rapidly, your hormones change again and you feel heavy with the weight of the baby. We know this sounds tough, but believe us it's worth it. In the meantime, here are some ways to support yourself through the first trimester fatigue:

Rest

It sounds simple, but how many of us actually let ourselves rest when we need to? Schedule times of rest with as much importance as you would food and hydration. Book out some evenings so that you can go to bed early, or at least collapse on the sofa with your feet up. If you start to give yourself a hard time, or feel like you are being lazy, remind yourself of everything that is happening inside you right now and then sit back down and reward your busy body with some rest so that it can do its job properly.

If you are navigating this journey solo, now could be a good time to bring in some extra support to allow you time to rest, just until those hormones settle a little and you feel like you have more energy.

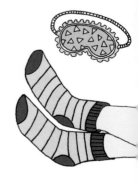

Get a good night's sleep

Some pregnant women are able to sleep at the drop of a hat, while others are exhausted but frustratingly completely unable to sleep. Pregnancy insomnia is thought to be hormone related (again), but can also be linked to anxiety, which is very common during pregnancy. Take a look at pages 80–84 for tips on getting more and better-quality sleep.

Get outside

Fresh air and gentle exercise can give us all an instant energy lift. We're often asked about what is safe when it comes to exercise during pregnancy, so see pages 37–38 for our advice and suggestions.

Eat and drink well

We go into more detail about nourishing grub for pregnancy on pages 28–36, but here are our top tips for eating and drinking to combat tiredness.

- Avoid caffeinated drinks and sugary, heavy foods. Although we are often tempted to reach for these to pick us up when we are tired, the energy they give us is short-lived, and can then make us feel even more tired when we come crashing back down again.

- Go for protein and carbohydrates, and slow-releasing energy foods such as bananas, oily fish (like salmon, sardines, mackerel and herring – although limit yourself to no more than two portions per week), brown rice, sweet potatoes, eggs, apples and dark chocolate.

- It's important to keep iron stores high in pregnancy. Increase your intake of iron-rich foods, which help with energy levels. You can find iron in meat, fish, green leafy veg, kidney beans, lentils, prunes and apricots.

- Stay hydrated – dehydration makes you tired and sluggish, so make sure you are drinking enough fluids.

Ask for help

Do ask for help. If you are so tired that you can't face going to work or looking after other children, then ask friends or family members to help. It's an honour to support a mum-to-be on her pregnancy journey and most people will be delighted to help you.

If your tiredness doesn't clear by the second trimester and you are still feeling exhausted, speak to your GP as they may want to run some tests and check you for low iron levels.

Point pressing

Acupressure is a form of alternative therapy in which manual pressure is applied, using fingers, to stimulate specific points on the body. DU20 (Bai Hui) is a fab acupressure point to stimulate for a boost of energy. To work the point:

1. Place both of your thumbs behind your ears, palms facing out to the front and your fingers pointing up (think bunny ears).

2. Now make your index fingers meet in the middle on top of your head and DU20 should be on the scalp under where your fingers meet. Press around and you will find a spot on the head that will feel more sensitive than the rest – that's DU20.

3. Press this spot for 30–60 seconds, close your eyes and take some deep breaths at the same time and you should feel energised in no time at all.

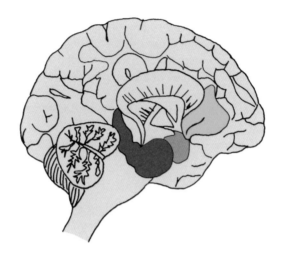

The Emotional Wobble

It is entirely normal for a positive pregnancy test to be accompanied by a whole array of raw emotions. These can initially feel quite erratic. You may be on cloud nine or perhaps you feel a little anxious until you have everything confirmed and are holding your little scan photo for evidence.

It is important to remember that there is no right or wrong response, and giving yourself time to process this news in whatever way feels right for you is essential. Whether your pregnancy was planned or not, whether it has happened much faster than you had anticipated, your pregnancy is the result of a fertility journey, you are a solo parent, or you are navigating pregnancy after loss, the bottom line is that however you arrived at this moment and whatever you are feeling, it's okay.

SUSPICIOUS MINDS!

If you're determined not to let the cat out of the bag then you might benefit from having a few responses up your sleeve ready for unwelcome questions.

HOW TO SHUT DOWN SUSPICIOUS QUESTIONING AT WORK

- You suffer with periods of insomnia and are sleeping badly at present, thus the eye bags.

- You have a UTI or ear infection and are on antibiotics.

- You are recovering from a migraine or stomach bug.

- If you have just arrived at work, you could say you suffer with travel sickness or motion sickness.

- You simply have a lot going on at home and are feeling slightly overwhelmed.

HOW TO SHUT DOWN QUESTIONING AT SOCIAL EVENTS

- Slyly buy yourself (or get someone in the know to buy you) a drink that looks like it could be an alcoholic beverage, such as a booze-free Bloody Mary, a non-alcoholic beer or the pregnancy classic: tonic with a slice of lemon.

- Say yes to the bubbles but keep hold of the one glass all evening, and you can just pretend it has been topped up.

- Be the designated driver as it's 'your turn'.

- Get your partner to also refrain from drinking if you are out together, and say you are both having a healthy eating / no drinking month.

- Turn down the booze and say you are still hungover from dinner with friends last night.

As well as arming yourself with quick comebacks and smothering your under-eyes with concealer the consistency of clotted cream, remember that if you are feeling unwell and bone-tired, there is no shame in slowing down.

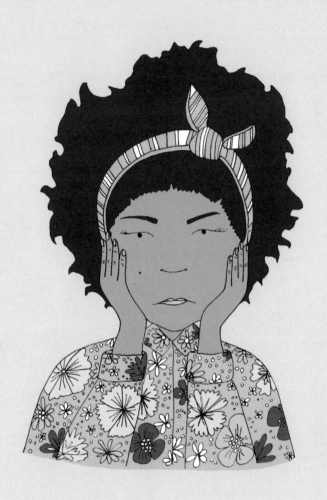

Green Around the Gills!

We know all too well that morning sickness is up there as one of the hardest side effects of pregnancy, affecting around 80 per cent of expectant mums. This name doesn't do it justice though, since you can feel sick at any time of the day or night. You may find the queasiness comes and goes during your pregnancy, or you may find you feel sick almost the entire time. Flick back to this section as often as you need for our top ten tips for coping with sickness:

1. **Eat little and often, and don't get hungry.** Eating little and often ensures that you do not overload your sensitive digestive system. Taking some crackers or biscuits (see page 23) to bed with you at night and having a quick snack in the morning before you get up can help reduce feelings of nausea. If you are up in the night for a wee and you can feel nausea creeping in, have a quick snack then settle back down to sleep.

2. **Know your triggers.** Identifying what makes your nausea worse can help you find ways to avoid these triggers where possible. This can often be the difference between feeling nauseous or actually vomiting. Feelings of sickness can be made worse by the following:

- Getting too hot
- Strong smells
- Bright lights
- Not drinking enough water (can be tricky if you are feeling sick, but see page 24 for ways to stay hydrated)
- Wearing tight-fitting waistbands or a tight bra, which is pressing on the top of your stomach
- Eating too much in one go and overloading your digestive system, or eating the wrong foods (see below)

3. **Foods to avoid and foods to eat.** Avoiding foods that are fatty, greasy, spicy or sugary is the best way to accommodate an overly sensitive digestive system. Don't worry too much about hitting your five-a-day right now – it's not uncommon for women to go off fruit and veg in the first trimester, and you will have plenty of vitamin stores to see you through, until you can stomach them again. For now, think comfort foods!

- Egg or avocado on toast
- Rice with some chicken and soy sauce (leave out the soy sauce if the smell is too strong and maybe add a little chicken stock instead)
- Clear broth or soup
- Pasta with a simple tomato sauce or just some grated cheese

Other foods that help with sickness

- Ginger any which way – freshly grated, chopped or as chews (available from health food shops) – can help.
- Or, make a mug of medicinal ginger tea by placing 2 tablespoons of peeled fresh root ginger chunks in a mug and pouring over some boiling water. Cover with a small plate or saucer and allow to steep for 5 minutes, then drink when cooled.
- Foods rich in vitamin B6, such as wholegrain wheat, seeds, nuts, avocados, spinach, bananas, papayas, fish, beans, lentils, chickpeas, prunes, raisins and apricots.

4. Perfect pongs. We are big fans of aromatherapy, but in the first trimester we think it's safest for you to use some natural pick-you-up pongs to settle your tummy and calm and uplift your mind. Slice a lemon and give it a good sniff – the scent of citrus is uplifting and very good for settling tummies. Or take a mint leaf and crush it between your fingers and rub it between your hands – mint is very refreshing and settling for nausea.

5. Carry a sick bag
The anxiety around being sick in public and 'making a scene' can often make you feel way worse than the actual sickness you are feeling. Anxiety increases stress hormones in your body and these make the symptoms feel more acute. Have some sick bags on you at all times, so that if you do need to be sick you can do so somewhere discreetly – or at least without making a mess.

6. nausea-busting juices

These wonderful juice recipes can help keep morning sickness at bay. Ask your partner to bring you a glass in the morning and drink it before you get out of bed. Alternatively, make one the night before and leave it in the fridge overnight to have when you get up. Try eating a couple of rice cakes or oatcakes with it, to give you a bit of energy to face the day. If the juice is too strong for you first thing in the morning, try drinking it around 11am or take it to work with you to sip at your desk.

You can also freeze these juices into ice lollies to suck on throughout the day to help ease nausea. Lollies can be a great way to keep fluids up if drinking makes you feel queasy. Pour them into an ice-lolly mould and place a lolly stick in each one and freeze overnight.

Paradiso:
Blitz: 1 peeled lime, 1 peeled and stoned ripe mango, ½ a peeled pineapple, 1 x 4cm chunk of peeled fresh root ginger, 150g live, low-fat yoghurt and a handful of ice cubes.

Ginger Juice-up:
Blitz: 1 x 4cm chuck of peeled fresh root ginger with ¼ large watermelon, skinned and deseeded. Pour in a glass over ice cubes and drink.

WONDROUS WATERMELON
Apart from being the best reminder to watch *Dirty Dancing* again, these beauties are full of nutrients and, at 92 per cent water, are perfect to help keep you hydrated. Watermelon can help ease heartburn and reduce swelling, its high-water content and fruit sugars can help alleviate morning sickness and, as it contains potassium, it can even help prevent muscle cramps.

---

7. ginger morning-sickness cookies

These cookies are a great snack to help keep you going when you really can't face anything else. If you feel too sick to even think about handling or preparing food, ask somebody to make some of these for you!

Makes 8–10 cookies

120g plain flour
120g coconut flour
1 tablespoon ground flaxseed
1 teaspoon bicarbonate of soda
a pinch of salt
2 teaspoons ground ginger
1 teaspoon ground cinnamon
1 tablespoon peeled and grated
  fresh root ginger
3 tablespoons caster sugar
1 teaspoon vanilla extract
2 medium eggs, beaten
2 tablespoons coconut oil,
  melted, plus extra for
  greasing
2 tablespoons molasses (or
  black treacle)

Preheat the oven to 180°C/160°C fan and grease a baking tray with a little coconut oil.

Mix all the dry ingredients and grated ginger together in a bowl.

Mix all the wet ingredients together in a separate bowl or jug, then combine with the dry ingredients to form a dough.

Put 8–10 dollops of the cookie mixture on the greased tray, spacing them out evenly so they're about 5cm apart.

Bake for 15–20 minutes, until golden brown, then remove from the oven and transfer to a wire rack and allow to cool. They will keep well in an airtight container for a few days – if they last that long!

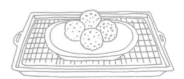

8. keep your fluids up

If you are being sick, you will need to make sure that you are replenishing your fluids to keep yourself hydrated. Sometimes, sipping plain water can make you feel nauseous, so adding a bit of flavour can make it more palatable, particularly if you have that horrible early-pregnancy metallic taste in your mouth. If you prefer a warm drink, peppermint, ginger and chamomile tea are all great for calming delicate tummies.

The Rehydration Ninja
This great coconut drink helps hydrate you quickly as it is full of electrolytes (natural salts and minerals), which are rehydration ninjas!

a thumb-sized chunk of
  fresh root ginger, peeled and
  finely grated
juice of ½ large lemon
juice of ½ orange
juice of ½ lime
700ml coconut water
2 teaspoons agave syrup or
  honey
¼ teaspoon salt
ice cubes, to serve

Put the ginger in a sieve over a bowl and squeeze out the juice using the back of a spoon. Discard the pulp, then mix the ginger juice with the lemon, orange and lime juices and the coconut water.

Stir in the agave syrup or honey and the salt.

Pour it over ice cubes in a glass and drink immediately, or store in the fridge for up to 24 hours and sip as required.

Note: you can also freeze this drink into ice lollies (see page 22) to suck on throughout the day whenever nausea strikes.

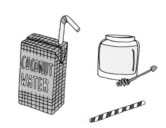

9. **Acupressure.** The acupressure point P6 (Nei-Kuan) is a fabulous point for combatting nausea, and is commonly used to treat travel sickness, which morning sickness can often feel like. You can stimulate the point manually with your finger, or you can wear some sea sickness bands. P6 pressure point can be found four finger-widths up from the edge of the hand in the middle of the wrist. Take some deep breaths while pressing into the point and you should start to feel the nausea settle after a minute or two.

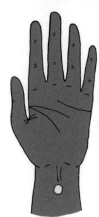

10. **Rest and relaxation**
Morning sickness will hit harder when you are tired or anxious, so it is even more important to build in time for rest and relaxation. See over the page for a calming breathing exercise – also, have a look at our yoga and breathing sequences on pages 39–41 and 140–143.

WHEN TO SEEK MORE SUPPORT
Although morning sickness is horrible, it is very common. However, 1 per cent of women suffer with a condition called hyperemesis gravidarum (HG) which causes extreme sickness and vomiting in pregnancy. It can be debilitating and needs careful treatment to keep mum and baby safe from dehydration. HG is not only physically hard, but can be mentally gruelling too, and many women will need lots of mental and emotional support. If you think you may be suffering with extreme sickness, ask your GP for help — there are safe medications nowadays that may help a little. A fabulous organisation for women with HG is www.pregnancysicknesssupport.org.com — it has a 24-hour helpline, offers a buddy system so you can talk to other women who have been through it and come out the other side, and has lots of further resources.

BREATHING EXERCISES FOR SICKNESS AND ANXIETY

Learning simple ways to control your breathing can be a game changer. Your brain and body are a brilliant partnership, always working together as a seamless feedback mechanism, with that grey matter of yours trying to respond appropriately to all these unusual physical sensations. Sometimes, however, it misinterprets these new physical experiences as unsafe or alarming, responding with an unhelpful dose of adrenaline, which can aggravate unpleasant pregnancy symptoms. Sometimes, all you can do if you are feeling overcome by nausea or anxiety is down tools, find a quiet place and take five minutes to calm down and soothe your overstimulated internal alarm system.

3 FLAMINGOS

Use this simple, soothing breathing tool any time to calm an anxious mind and help reduce nausea.

1. Find a comfortable place to sit, or lie on your side if sitting up exaggerates any unwelcome physical sensations. Close your eyes.

2. Relax your shoulders down (you may find rotating them backwards then forwards helps release any tension).

3. Drop/hang your head slightly, especially if you are feeling nauseous or dizzy.

4. Place one hand splayed out across your tummy, above your belly button and below your chest.

5. Breathe in for 3 seconds through your nose. For a sense of pace, think 'one flamingo, two flamingos, three flamingos', in your own natural rhythm.

6. Feel your hand being pushed away slowly and gently by that inhalation, and the side of your ribs expand, like you are inflating an invisible balloon inside yourself.

7. Breathe out of your mouth for 6 calm, controlled seconds (at the same pace as your in-breaths).

8. Repeat at least three times and then reassess how you are feeling.

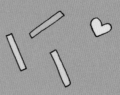

'Pregnancy sickness is rotten, like feeling hungover, but without any of the fun the night before. It also makes you do weird stuff! I remember a time when I was halfway through my spag bol dinner, and a wave of nausea came over me and I had to throw up into a bowl at the dinner table (eek!).

This funnily enough didn't bother me too much – what did bother me was my husband taking away my dinner that I hadn't finished yet, assuming I wouldn't want it anymore. The thing about morning sickness is that once you've puked, you actually feel rather good after – and well up for finishing your dinner!'

BELINDA, MUM OF TWO

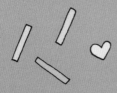

Nourishing Grub: Part 1

Our general rule of thumb for the first trimester is eat what you can stomach! Saying that, there are some foods to avoid and indeed some foods that you should try to include to make sure you are getting enough nutrients. We've listed these below as an easy reference.

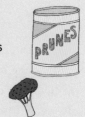

Things to avoid ....

- Soft blue cheese and soft mould-ripened cheese (cheeses with a white rind, like brie and camembert), as these can contain the listeria bacteria. You can eat hard cheeses and non mould-ripened soft cheeses, like feta, mozzarella, ricotta and halloumi.

- Raw or undercooked eggs - although if they have a British Lion Code stamp on them, they are produced under strict food safety standards and are considered very low risk for salmonella and safe to eat undercooked. So if you want a dippy egg and soldiers, just look for eggs with the British Lion Code stamp.

- Paté and any raw or undercooked meat has a risk of salmonella and toxoplasmosis. All meat should be well cooked, with only clear juices coming from it (no blood).

- Cold-cured meats such as salami, prosciutto and chorizo carry the risk of the listeria bacteria. You can reduce the risk of parasites by freezing the meat for 4 days at home before eating it.

- Liver, or products containing liver, as it has too much vitamin A in it.

- Game meat, such as rabbit, pheasant, goose, duck and venison. These may contain lead from the lead pellets.

- Be careful with fish - no shark, marlin or swordfish. Limit your tuna to two steaks and no more than four tins a week, as it can contain high levels of mercury. Limit oily fish, such as sardines, salmon and mackerel, to no more than two portions a week as they can contain pollutants.

- Sushi - but you can eat sushi if the fish has been frozen first. Ask if you're not sure.

- Raw shellfish - only eat cooked shellfish.

- Raw unpasteurised milk and dairy products - unpasteurised dairy can contain microbes that can upset our tummies and also carries a risk of listeria.

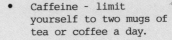

- Caffeine - limit yourself to two mugs of tea or coffee a day.

- Alcohol - it is advised that you do not drink any alcohol during your pregnancy.

Things to include ....

CALCIUM
During pregnancy you need calcium for the development of baby's bones, teeth, heart, nerves and muscles. The best source of calcium is dairy, but you can also find it in green leafy veg, sardines (with the bones), almonds, fortified cereals and fortified plant milks.

FIBRE
Essential for a healthy digestive system, and especially helpful in pregnancy to avoid constipation. Do remember to add more fluid to your diet if you increase your fibre intake. Eat plenty of fresh fruit and veg, lentils and wholegrain cereals.

FOLATE
Folic acid is important for the healthy development of your baby, and can significantly reduce the chance of neural tube defects. Although it is a good idea to increase your intake of folate-rich foods, it is very tricky to get the dosage you need from food alone and this is why a folic acid supplement is recommended until twelve weeks (see page 31 for

more on supplements). Green leafy vegetables, brown rice, granary bread and fortified breakfast cereals are some of the best food sources.

IODINE
Iodine is important for healthy brain development in your baby. Eat tuna (see page 29 for how much tuna you should eat each week), eggs, butter beans and prunes.

IRON
Your body needs higher stores of iron during pregnancy to make extra blood for you and your baby. Being low in iron can cause anaemia and make you feel tired and unwell, so it's a good idea to include a couple of portions of iron-rich food in your diet each day. Iron-rich foods include meat, fish, eggs, green leafy veg, kidney beans, prunes, apricots and baked potatoes with the skin on. See pages 14-15 for more on being low in iron.

MAGNESIUM
This is important for bone and muscle health, calcium absorption, and supporting a good metabolism, and is a great help for soothing cramps and restless leg syndrome. It can also help with symptoms of anxiety. Good food sources include wholewheat bread or pasta, brown rice, oats, quinoa, spinach, almonds, cashews and peanuts, dark chocolate, black beans and avocado.

POTASSIUM
Good for muscle health and reduces blood pressure and water retention. Eat plenty of fruit and veg, including bananas, oranges, cantaloupe melon, apricots, grapefruit, spinach, broccoli, potatoes, sweet potatoes, peas and cucumber.

PROTEIN
Protein is an important building block for bones, muscles, cartilage, skin and blood, as well as being used to make enzymes and hormones, so you can see how important it is for us to have enough in our diet. In pregnancy, especially, we need protein to repair and build tissues. Eat plenty of lean meats, beans, pulses, tempeh, nuts, fish and eggs.

VITAMIN C
Protects cells and helps keep them healthy. It also assists many of the body's functions including the formation of collagen, maintaining a good immune system, wound healing and the absorption of iron, and

it helps keep cartilage, bones and teeth healthy. Eat oranges, green leafy veg, peppers, berries, kiwi fruit, tomatoes and peas.

VITAMIN D

This clever vitamin regulates the amount of calcium and phosphate your body absorbs, helping to keep bones, teeth and muscles healthy. It also helps keep your immune system functioning at optimum levels. Get out in the sun for 15 minutes each day, or find vitamin D in all oily fish (no more than two portions per week), cheese, eggs, fortified plant milks and fortified cereals.

ZINC

Zinc supports your baby's development, playing an important role in the construction of your baby's cells, DNA and tissue growth. It can also help us cope with stress and keep energy on an even keel. Find it in - among other things - beef, lamb, pumpkin seeds and ginger.

SUPPLEMENTS

Do make sure that you are taking your pregnancy vitamins. It is recommended that you take 400mg folic acid each day until you are twelve weeks pregnant. The Department of Health and Social Care also advises taking a vitamin D supplement. Do not take vitamin A or any supplements containing vitamin A (retinol) as too much could harm your baby. It is always best to seek the guidance of a nutritional therapist if you are thinking about adding any other supplements to your diet during pregnancy.

recipes ~ smoothies

Smoothies are especially great when you are queasy and feel like you can't stomach a whole meal. As they are already blended, your digestive system won't have to work too hard to process them. They are also a great way of getting a hit of nourishment without spending ages in the kitchen, which can hold far too many food smells in one place for an upset tummy and sensitive nose. You can even pre-prepare your smoothie ingredients and freeze them in individual containers, so then you literally only have to chuck the contents into your blender and add some liquid! If you are really struggling, ask somebody to prepare the freezer packs for you.

We've kept our smoothie recipes as simple as possible – just chuck everything in a blender, add the liquid and blitz! If you prefer your smoothies cold, add a handful of ice cubes before or after the blitzing process, but remember the colder it is, the harder it is to digest. A room temperature smoothie will be gentler on the digestive process.

Morning Sickness-settling
1 banana, peeled
120g oats
1 teaspoon peeled and grated
   fresh root ginger
1 pear, cored, peeled and sliced
1 tablespoon chia seeds
½ teaspoon ground turmeric
   (optional – leave it out if you
   don't like the taste)
1 tablespoon maple syrup
250ml drinking coconut milk

Constipation-easing
1 apple, cored, peeled and cut
   into chunks
1 carrot, peeled and cut into
   chunks
3 dates, stones removed
3 prunes, stones removed
a handful of spinach
1 tablespoon ground flaxseed
200ml pineapple juice
200ml drinking coconut milk

Calming

¼ pineapple, peeled and cut into chunks
½ orange, peeled
1 peeled, frozen banana (slice the banana into chunks before you freeze it)
2 plums, stones removed
½ teaspoon edible lavender flowers
1 tablespoon ground flaxseed
200ml drinking coconut milk

Insomnia-busting

8–10 juicy cherries (fresh or frozen), stones removed
1 banana, peeled
2 tablespoons honey
½ teaspoon freshly grated or ground nutmeg
250ml milk of your choice

Energy-boosting

juice of 1 orange
juice of ½ lemon
¼ watermelon, peeled and cut into chunks
1 mango, peeled and stone removed
1 banana, peeled
2 fresh mint leaves
250ml coconut water

Iron-rich

a handful of spinach
juice of 1 orange
2 fresh apricots, stones removed
1 tablespoon ground flaxseed
a handful of fresh or frozen raspberries
½ avocado, peeled and stoned
2 dates, stones removed
250ml drinking coconut milk

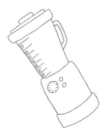
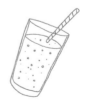

quick and easy snacks for bone-tired mamas-to-be and queasy tummies

<u>Loaded toast</u>

We love toast and we know lots of our mamas do, too. It is super-comforting when you are feeling a bit tired or queasy. Plus, even better, it's really easy to make. But don't forget that you can top your toast with more than just your usual spreads for some quick and easy goodness. Try some of the following:

- Peanut butter and banana and/or a scattering of pomegranate seeds
- Smashed avocado and scrambled egg (add some tinned mackerel if you fancy a little something extra)
- Marmite and baked beans (don't knock it until you've tried it!). Add a poached egg for an extra dose of protein
- Sautéed mushroom and tomatoes
- Grilled cheese and sautéed onion
- Hummus, cucumber and black olives
- Halloumi, rocket and roasted tomatoes from a jar
- Ricotta, figs, honey and walnuts
- Chocolate spread, strawberries and chopped hazelnuts

<u>Energy Balls</u>

Pregnancy tiredness or not, we all hit a mid-afternoon slump when we reach for the biscuits now and then, don't we? These energy balls are a fab way of giving ourselves that sweet hit and energy boost without a packet of digestives in sight! They are great if you are feeling queasy and don't fancy eating much, but can manage a nibble and a cuppa. Energy balls can be made in bulk and kept in the freezer for up to 3 months, so you can make up a store to keep you going. Just defrost them in the fridge. They are a fab snack during labour, too.

You can pretty much use anything you like in them, but we've given you a basic recipe below along with a few ideas for how to 'pimp your balls'!

Makes 8–12 balls

2 handfuls of almonds
2 handfuls of pecans
2 handfuls of stoned dates
1 handful of dried apricots (go for the unsulphured ones)
2 tablespoons ground flaxseed
2 tablespoons melted coconut oil
1 tablespoon maple syrup
2 tablespoons peanut butter
a few tablespoons of cacao powder, desiccated coconut or chia seeds, to coat (optional)

Blitz the nuts to a fine crumb, then add the rest of the ingredients (except the coating option) and blitz again until a sticky mixture forms – add more syrup if needed.

Scrape the mixture out and use your hands to roll it into 8–12 even-sized balls (about the size of a golf ball), then roll each ball in a coating of your choice.

Try adding the following ingredients to the food processor in your basic mix. Don't be afraid play around with flavours – the possibilities are endless!

- Dark chocolate chips
- Goji berries
- Chopped fresh root ginger
- Matcha powder
- Spices – ground cinnamon, freshly grated or ground nutmeg
- Raisins
- Crushed pretzels
- Popcorn
- Vanilla extract
- Lemon or orange juice or zest
- Poppy seeds

warm up your salads

The body has to work harder to digest cold foods because we have to warm the food internally first, before the digestive process can start. This can be hard work on a sensitive or tired tummy, so we suggest trying to eat more warm than cold food if you are feeling a bit delicate. That said, you do lose some nutrients in the cooking process, especially boiling (if you are pouring the liquid away) so opt for sautéing, baking or steaming and avoid overcooking – the crunchier the veg, the more vitamins are still inside!

Here's our favourite, comforting warm salad, packed with nutrients, but play around and make it your own – the options are endless. If you would prefer a vegan option, try adding 200g of warm lentils, or 250g sautéed mushrooms in place of the salmon.

Warm Salmon Salad

Serves 2

2 salmon fillets
olive oil
1 large sweet potato, peeled and
  cut into chunks
125g green beans
70g broccoli
2 tomatoes, chopped
a generous handful of rocket
salt and pepper

Preheat the oven to 180°C/160°C fan. Place the salmon fillets on a lightly oiled baking tray, skin-side down.

Add the sweet potato chunks, drizzle with olive oil and season with salt and pepper.

Bake in the oven for 20–30 minutes, turning the sweet potato chunks over halfway through.

Meanwhile, steam the green beans and broccoli.

Serve the salmon and sweet potato with the chopped tomatoes on a bed of rocket, with the greens alongside.

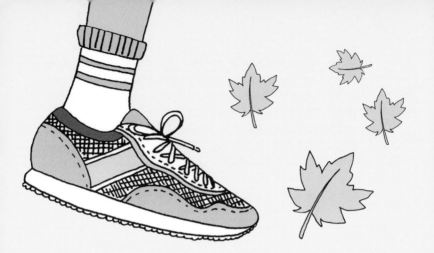

Keep on Moving!

We get asked a lot if it's safe to exercise in pregnancy and the short answer is yes. Exercise improves your muscle tone and strength, which can make it easier for you to adapt to the changes that pregnancy brings (and also help prepare you for labour and recovery after the birth). That said, there are a few provisos that you should adhere to, so that you ensure you are exercising safely.

- **Your normal is okay.** It's best not to start any new high-impact exercise or health regime in early pregnancy, when your body is already working hard. If you are an active person already, then continue as normal but do let your instructor know you are pregnant (if you attend fitness classes or go to the gym) and follow their advice. If you generally do very little exercise, then you may benefit from some gentle walking, swimming, pregnancy yoga or pregnancy Pilates to keep the body strong and supple – but do start gently and build up gradually.

- **Listen to your body!** If you feel fit and well then exercise has lots of health- and mood-boosting benefits for mums-to-be. Lots of women, however, feel too sick and tired in the first trimester, choosing not to exercise and instead opting to rest in the early stages. This can be the case in the last trimester too, when some women feel too heavy and tired. This is perfectly okay – your body knows best.

- **Go at your own pace.** It is important to move and keep that circulation going, but find an exercise that feels comfortable. Remember, we all experience pregnancy differently, so don't try to keep up with your mate's exercise regime; stick to one that suits you!

- **Watch your pelvis.** Hypermobility in the pelvis can be a side effect of those wonderful pregnancy hormones, so keep an eye on any exercises that put too much stretch and strain in that area. Avoid squatting, lunging or yoga postures that are too opening in the pelvis. Mention to your instructor if you have any pelvic pain; there will always be an adaptation of the exercise that you can do instead. For example – if you are experiencing groin pain in pregnancy, avoid breaststroke legs while swimming.

- **Hit the water.** During the second and especially the third trimester, when ligaments are loose and your bump is heavy, aqua natal classes can be a great way to exercise, as you can enjoy the buoyancy of water which takes the weight off your joints, making the exercise have a lower impact.

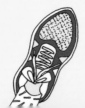
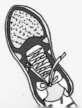

yoga for pregnancy

We are big fans of pregnancy yoga! It gives you a brilliant opportunity to take time out of your busy day, calm your mind and breath and to connect with your baby. We asked one of our favourite yoga teachers, Kiranjot (a doula and kundalini yoga teacher), for some simple but super-helpful yoga practices to use whenever you feel the need to ease an ache or calm a worry. Yoga is also a fantastic way to encourage baby into an optimum position for birth and teaches you practical ways to manage the intensity of labour.

A few common-sense things for keen yogis to know:

- Do not put awkward pressure on your uterus.

- No deep twists or back bends.

- No double leg lifts or sit-ups.

- Avoid straining or over-stretching your pelvis if you are suffering from any pain in the hips or groin (mention this to your teacher who can help you adapt the positions).

- Do not push yourself so hard you get short of breath.

- In the first trimester it's common to feel a bit like a zombie as you grow your baby and all its organs, so listen to your body and do not work it hard when you're tired. Rest is best.

Sitali Pranayam

This is a brilliant cooling and soothing breath, great if you are feeling hot and bothered. An aid for your digestion, it's also worth trying if you are suffering from morning sickness or heartburn.

- Roll your tongue like a straw. Suck your breath in through the mouth. If you can't roll your tongue, suck your breath in through the teeth instead.

- Exhale through the nose.

- You will feel a cool in-breath straight away, but continue for at least 3 minutes for full effect.

Spinal flexes

Reduces brain fog, releases tension from the shoulders and opens up the chest so you can breathe more deeply. These flexes are great at any stage in your pregnancy. Do them cross-legged and pull on the front ankle to really move the spine, in a chair if getting to the floor is difficult, or do them standing up, with your hands braced on your thighs to really get the hips moving. Later in pregnancy, do them on your hands and knees – known as cat-cow (see page 64) – to help encourage baby into an optimal position for birth.

- If seated, keep your head level and eyes closed.

- Inhale, and as you do, start to flex the spine forwards like an 'S', pushing your chest out forwards too.

- Push your shoulders down and back by squeezing your shoulder blades together as you come forward.

- As you begin to exhale, flex the spine back, curling like a 'C'.

- Breathe long and slow, deep, equal breaths in time with your movements. Listen to each breath.

- Take your time to learn to follow your breath so you are perfectly synchronised with each movement.

- Continue for at least 3 minutes.

PLEASE NOTE:
If you have any pain in your pelvis do tell your yoga teacher or seek advice from a qualified women's health osteopath / chiropractor. You may be advised to avoid certain poses that could cause you further discomfort. Also see pages 49—52.

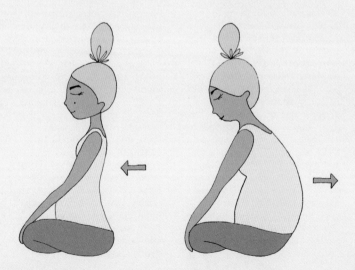

UP CLOSE AND PERSONAL

Some women may not have been to the hospital or even visited their doctor very much until they became pregnant. Now it feels like you're there sharing personal information, giving blood and talking about boobs and vaginas on a weekly basis. We understand that there will no doubt be moments when you feel a little embarrassment creep in or feel a little vulnerable, but remember that your health professionals see women every single day and they are there to check you and baby are healthy and give you the information you need to feel calm and supported.

PRIVATE CONVERSATIONS

All conversations with your health professional are confidential, unless they need to refer you to other professionals to support you further. Do not be alarmed if, at your booking appointment with a midwife, she asks you about your complete medical history including your mental health, family relationships, sexual health and whether you have ever experienced domestic violence. As intrusive as this may feel coming from a complete stranger, know that every pregnant woman will discuss these topics during their initial appointment and at certain check-in meetings along the way.

EXTERNAL PHYSICAL CONTACT

During your visits to see midwives and doctors you are likely to experience physical contact, whether this be taking your blood pressure, palpating your tummy to feel the position of your little one, or using a tape measure to chart growth. Your midwife will explain what she or he is doing and ask consent before touching you. If modesty is important to you, wear comfortable clothing where you can have easy access to your upper arm and tummy. Don't rock up in a jumpsuit that means you have to strip down to your waist and feel more exposed than necessary - unless you don't care!

INTERNAL PHYSICAL CONTACT

It is very likely that, at some point during your pregnancy, you will have a vaginal examination. Your midwives and doctors do this day in, day out, and will know how to make you feel as comfortable as possible. We encourage you to be assertive and always ask questions as to why, when and how any examination will take place before giving your consent. If it will make you more comfortable, ask for a chaperone to be present and, if necessary, tell them you need them to stop for a moment.

TRIGGERING INTERACTIONS

If you have a history of any intimate violation or sexual abuse, please do make your care providers aware. This will be discussed during your booking and a subtle sticker or code is likely to be placed on the front of your maternity notes. However, sometimes these notes can be missed so please do remind whoever is caring for you so that they can be even more aware and gentle with how vulnerable you may be feeling.

NEEDLE PHOBIA

Nobody loves having their blood taken, but having a fear of needles can feel particularly difficult during pregnancy and birth. We understand the extreme physical responses a phobia can present, so here are some self-soothing techniques that we have used over the years.

- Write that you have a needle phobia on the front page of your maternity notes to alert your health provider.
- Prepare yourself by applying EMLA numbing cream to the appropriate area an hour before your blood test.
- Take someone with you who can offer a hand to hold.
- Ask to lie down if you know a blood test is likely to make you feel lightheaded or faint.
- Let your care provider know that you do not want to have them talk through the procedure with you if it is likely to make you feel worse.
- Press on the acupressure point P6 as shown on page 25 to help with anxiety and nausea prior to and following any needle use.
- Practise the 3 Flamingos breath on page 26.

What if it's Not My First Baby?

This may not be your first rodeo, but remember each pregnancy is unique! You'll be amazed how differently we can carry our babies and how varied our emotional experience can be depending on the hormones and life situations playing out each time. But there are a few fundamental differences that you will notice if this isn't your first baby:

- You may be surprised by a bump suddenly appearing out of nowhere and much earlier than last time. This can be a little tricky if you are trying to keep your pregnancy a secret until you've had your first scan, so you may have to get clever with your clothes. This happens because your muscles are likely to be a bit looser, but also because muscle memory allows muscle fibres to give much more quickly this time around. The good news is that you may suffer less with stretching pains than you did in your first pregnancy.

- If you suffered with pelvic girdle pain (PGP), symphysis pubis dysfunction (SPD) (see page 50) or instability in your first pregnancy, it will often occur earlier in your second. This is generally caused by an earlier release of the hormone relaxin, which helps to soften your ligaments in order to allow room for your baby to grow. The trick here is to nip it in the bud as soon as you feel any symptoms. See our section on pelvic health on pages 49–52 for lots of tips on treating and supporting pelvic instability.

- If this isn't your first baby, you may need to be more inventive at carving out time to rest. If your little one naps after lunch, make sure you nap with them whenever you can, or go to bed when they do in the evening and have a lovely early night. And don't be afraid to call in help if the tiredness hits and you need an extra pair of hands.

- Your pelvic floor may be more sensitive, or feel a little weaker, especially if you are having your littles close together, or if you had any pelvic floor issues the first time. Be extra good at doing your pelvic floor exercises – set reminders on your phone, or using a pelvic floor reminder app. See our pelvic health section on pages 49–52.

- You may feel more Braxton Hicks (practice contractions) in your second and third trimester than you did last time. Our body is a remarkable thing, and this happens for two reasons. First, it comes down to those muscle memory receptors again. Secondly, it can be our body's way of slowing us down and stopping us from overdoing it. Research suggests that we may experience more Braxton Hicks when we are doing too much, so if you feel like you are experiencing more than the usual, try putting your feet up and resting for a while and they should settle down.

> Note: If your Braxton Hicks continue to come often, speak to your midwife or GP as this can also be a sign of a urine infection.

- No doubt at some point in this pregnancy you'll sit down with a cuppa feeling reflective and hugely emotional, wondering about how you will ever love another baby like the one(s) you already have. We'll let you in on a secret … there is SO much love inside there, and with each new baby, the store cupboard opens up and a whole new order of love arrives. Everything will be okay!

WORD TO YOUR PARTNER

Congratulations, you are also having a baby! You are going to play a very important role throughout this whole pregnancy and birth journey and have the ability to bring comfort and support like no other. It can be easy to feel like a passenger right now, as your partner is going through the day-to-day physical and mental highs and lows of the first trimester, but know that you can make the hugest difference with the simplest nurturing gestures. Remember: you are a team from Day One of the pregnancy, birth and parenting journey.

HOW TO BE THE 'PERFECT PARTNER' IN THE FIRST TRIMESTER

- Remind them how loved and gorgeous they are despite the nausea, exhaustion, tender boobs and wild pregnancy hormones.

- Understand that she is not being irrational: there is a rapid increase in oestrogen and progesterone hormones in the first trimester that can cause high emotions and mood swings (see page 10).

- Bring her a nausea-quenching smoothie (see pages 32-33) or a peppermint tea and dry crackers in the morning before she gets out of bed, to help her start her day well.

- Don't take a chippy comment personally, as she may be less patient and more anxious than usual - remind her that she is not alone and that you are there to support her too!

- Remember that when she says she is tired not to answer 'yeah, me too', but understand that she is referring to the sort of fatigue that physically hurts, as so much energy is going into growing a mini human.

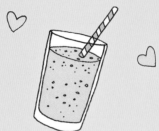

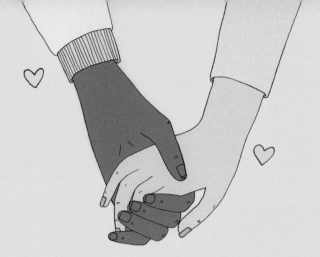

- Be sensitive when she dry-heaves after opening the fridge, dishwasher or washer-dryer. No, she is not being dramatic: pregnancy hormones can make women ultra-sensitive to smells and tastes.

- Prepare or batch-cook food for the two of you when possible.

- Offer to nip out late to get those weird and wonderful food cravings that she is desperate for. 'Pickled onions and Coco Pops? Got it.'

- Know that when she's venting about how rotten she feels, she's not asking you to fix it, but just that she needs you to listen and offer up some TLC.

- Be sensitive, patient and calm with her as she adjusts mentally and physically to pregnancy.

- Don't worry, this period of time is short in the grand scheme of things and is likely to begin to settle as she transitions into her second trimester at twelve weeks.

- If in doubt, offer up a foot rub (see our massage section on pages 100-104 for more details). This will help relax her, connect you both physically, and calm her anxieties.

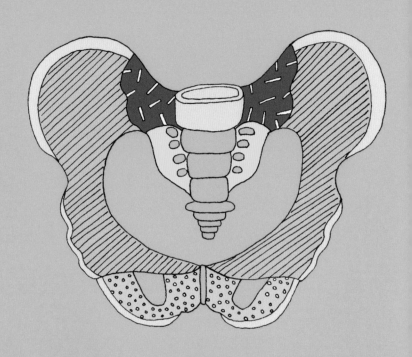

Pelvic Health

As your baby grows, your body has to adapt and change to accommodate it, increasing the production of relaxin, oestrogen and progesterone hormones to allow for your soft tissues to stretch and change shape. Sometimes, with all these changes, you may experience some discomfort or pain, but please rest assured that most of the time these problems can be easily treated. Remember that with pelvic issues, prevention is definitely better than cure. Here are our top tips for supporting your pelvis throughout pregnancy:

1. **Check your sleeping set-up.** Making sure you are supporting your hips while you sleep is so important to prevent pressure pain, or glute and hip pain from sleeping in a side-lying position. A soft mattress topper and a pillow or two between your knees is key!

2. **Stay active.** Keeping mobile (as long as this doesn't make the pain worse) is important to keep the muscles well-nourished and strong. Too much inactivity causes the blood circulation to slow down, causing tight, achy muscles.

3. **Limit sofa time.** Sitting on a sofa isn't great for most people's back and pelvis, but especially so for all you pregnant mamas. If you are watching TV, swap between the sofa, sitting on a birthing ball, or even lying on your side with your pillow between your knees.

4. **See a physio.** A women's health physio can check you out properly and find out what is causing the pain. They will then show you stretches you can do at home to keep the pain at bay. You can get a referral to a physio from your GP. And don't forget all the lovely massage sections in this book, which will help keep the surrounding muscles nice and healthy (see pages 100–104, and 182–183).

5. **Watch your posture.** If your groin is getting twingey and you are getting the sensation many of our ladies refer to as 'fanny daggers', you may need to support your symphysis a little better (the little ligament in the bottom-centre of the pelvis, by your pubic bone). Keeping knees and ankles together, and avoiding standing on one leg to put your pants on, will really help to reduce inflammation and ease the stabbing pains. We always say, 'Think Short Skirt, No Knickers'! When you move, imagine you are wearing a short skirt with no pants: think about how

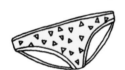 you would naturally keep your knees and ankles together and this is exactly how you'll need to be moving to support the pubis better.

Symphysis Pubis Dysfunction (SPD)

This condition is caused by the ligaments between the two sides of your pubic bones becoming looser, causing too much movement and making the pelvis unstable. If you are experiencing pelvic discomfort, visit your GP and ask for a referral to a physio which they can do via your local hospital, or visit your local private women's health physio. The key here is to nip it in the bud as soon as you can, so don't wait until it's really bad before you get seen.

Know Your Pelvic Floor

Tina Mason BSc (Hons), HCPC, MCSP, MAACP, MPOGP, Women's Health Brighton (sister clinic to Brighton Physiotherapy Clinic) gives us the pelvic low-down:

Your pelvic floor is a group of muscles that sits like a hammock, lining the bottom of your pelvis. Unfortunately, with pregnancy hormones allowing your soft tissues to become stretchier and the weight of your baby pressing down onto your pelvic floor, these muscles may become weakened and stretched throughout your pregnancy.

Urinary leakage in pregnancy is common but the good news is that there are lots of ways to prevent it. Starting pelvic floor muscle training as early as possible can help you avoid this and stave off problems postnatally, too. If the first time you think about your pelvic floor is after having your baby, it is much harder to work the muscles as they will have been stretched and weakened, whereas if you train them throughout pregnancy, it will be easier for you to engage with them afterwards, assisting in the decrease of incontinence and helping to speed recovery to your pelvic area.

Here are some tips on how to train your pelvic floor muscles:

- Find a comfortable position where you can relax and concentrate. This can be lying down or relaxed sitting.

- The breath is an important factor in carrying out your pelvic floor contractions correctly: start by taking a few big, deep belly breaths to help you relax.

- Take another breath in and as you breathe out, try to zip up (contract) your pelvic floor from anus to pubis. The action is the same as trying to stop yourself passing wind or stopping yourself going for a wee.

- Hold this contraction and try to breathe normally for a count of 10. If you feel you cannot hold it for that long, don't panic. Take a few more big belly breaths to relax and try again. At first, you may only be able to hold the contraction for a couple of seconds a couple of times before you feel it gets tired, but that's okay and with practice this will improve.

- The relaxation phase is just as important as the contraction, so take your time to breathe in fully and as you do so, really let go of all tension from the muscles, releasing fully.

- The aim is to be able to hold the contraction for 10 seconds, 10 times with a full relaxation of the muscle in between.

- It is also good to train the fast-twitch fibres that kick in when you laugh, cough or sneeze to prevent you from leaking during these actions. Start by taking a big breath in, then on your out-breath squeeze your pelvic floor muscles. Take another breath in to relax the muscle, then squeeze again on an out-breath. Repeat this 10 times.

Vaginal Health

We all know our tummy and breasts will expand in pregnancy, we expect achy backs and weird cravings, but how many of us enter pregnancy knowing about the changes that happen down below? Knowing what changes to expect helps us to understand the difference between normal changes to our bits and when we might need to visit our GP or midwife for some advice.

Get to know yourself. It's a really good idea to have a proper look 'down there' before your bump gets too big and you can no longer see past your belly! Knowing what your vagina looks like and what your 'normal' is can be really helpful in identifying changes in pregnancy and postnatally. We often get women to have a look at their vaginas in the postnatal period to reassure them that all is well, and we are so surprised by how many women have never had a good look. Your vagina is amazing! It's such an important part of who we are. Go on, grab a mirror and take a peek.

So, what should we expect? Vaginal discharge. Higher levels of oestrogen and progesterone, as well as an increase in blood volume and flow to the vagina, causes an increase in vaginal discharge. Normal pregnancy discharge is generally thin and watery or white and milky. It may well thicken and increase in volume as your pregnancy progresses. If you find it is wetting through your pants, wear panty liners, but do choose an unperfumed range, otherwise these may cause irritation. Although your discharge will have an odour, it shouldn't smell bad or have a colour to it.

Vaginal dryness. It is not uncommon to experience some vaginal dryness during pregnancy, especially in the first and third trimesters when oestrogen and progesterone levels fluctuate sharply. You may find using a lube or unscented vaginal moisturiser will help – buy a non-perfumed, organic brand. Most commercial branded lubes are full of scents and chemicals and will almost certainly leave you feeling irritated.

Swollen labia and vagina. Increased blood flow to the vagina means it is not unusual for your labia and vagina to appear swollen and feel fuller. It may also cause them to darken and take on a bluish tint. On the plus side, this swelling and increased blood flow may also increase sensitivity – which can increase your libido and make you feel more easily aroused.

Vulva varicose veins. These are the same blue raised veins you may have seen on people's legs, and are caused by pressure on the veins from the extra blood flow. Although nothing to worry about, a vulva varicose vein can feel full and uncomfortable, creating a feeling of pressure. This can be relieved by regularly using cooling maternity pads (see pages 120–121) to reduce inflammation. Also try regular sitz baths (see page 56). Most go away on their own several weeks after birth, but see your GP if you are concerned.

CALL YOUR MIDWIFE OR GP IF YOU HAVE ANY OF THE FOLLOWING:
- Unpleasant-smelling discharge
- Discharge that is green or yellow
- Your urine smells and is cloudy
- You have pain when you pass urine
- You feel itchy or sore around or inside your vagina
- You are experiencing any vaginal blood loss

Yeast Infections

Yeast infections usually occur when there has been a change to the normal pH levels in the vagina. Symptoms of a yeast infection include vaginal itching, a thick white discharge that smells yeasty, and a hot burning sensation in and around the vagina. If you have thrush, you can visit the GP to get some medicated treatment, but here are our Top Ten natural ways to soothe the irritation and prevent it from reoccurring.

- **Do** make some of the cooling maternity pads on pages 120–121. Use them to take the inflammation and heat out of the vulva – this is so soothing and helps stop the itching.

- **Do** wear cotton underwear and avoid synthetic materials, which encourage heat and moisture retention, providing the perfect breeding ground for candida.

- **Do** change pads regularly if you are wearing them, and use organic and unperfumed pads if possible. Better still, these days you can buy bamboo washable panty liners – better for your bits and the environment!

- **Do** always wipe front to back after using the loo. And avoid perfumed toilet paper.

- **Do** go commando! When you are home, try to go pants-free and allow the air to circulate around your bits. This is easily done by wearing a skirt and no knickers.

- **Do** remember that good-old natural yoghurt can help too! The acidophilus bacteria, which is what helps get rid of thrush, is quite a low dose, so it's not great at it, but it is very soothing. Try inserting yoghurt into the vagina for a cooling relief – but wear a pad, or if you are airing your vagina, lie on a towel, as the yoghurt will eventually come out, and you don't want it all over the sheets.

- **Don't** use perfumed detergent to wash your underwear – use a detergent designed for sensitive skin.

- **Don't** wear tight-fitting clothes, as this also creates a warm environment for bacterial and yeast growth.

- **Don't** use anything strong and scented when washing or bathing. This will affect the pH levels in your vagina and exacerbate the symptoms you may already have.

- **Don't** eat too much sugar – this includes fresh and dried fruits. Thrush thrives on a sugary diet, so try cutting sugar out of your diet for a while to help keep it at bay.

SITZ BATH
A great way to treat, prevent and soothe the symptoms of thrush and infections. Repeat as often as you need, but at least twice a day.

1. Place 3 chamomile tea bags in a large jug, add boiling water and steep for 30 minutes.
2. Run a shallow bath (no higher than thigh height).
3. Add 2 drops of tea tree essential oil to 1 cup of Epsom salts, and add to the bath.
4. Pour in the chamomile tea and give it a good swirl to mix it all up. You can also add a cup of apple cider vinegar, which can help settle pH levels.
5. Sit in the shallow bath for at least 10–15 minutes. You can stay in it for as long as you like: if it gets chilly, just add some extra hot water.
6. When you get out, gently pat yourself dry with a clean towel and either put on some clean cotton knickers or go commando and let the air circulate!

Urinary Tract Infections (UTIs)

UTIs are more common in pregnancy due to the internal changes in the urinary tract. The uterus sits on top of the bladder and, as it grows in size and weight, it can press down and block the effective drainage of urine from the bladder, causing infection.

Symptoms of a UTI are:
- Pain or burning when peeing
- Needing to wee more often than usual
- Smelly or cloudy pee
- Pain in your lower tummy
- Blood in your pee
- Feeling tired or unwell

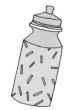

UTIs can be treated safely with antibiotics during pregnancy, so visit your doctor for treatment. Here are some top tips to help ease the symptoms and prevent reoccurrence of infection:

- Up your water intake (aim for 6–8 glasses a day) and be sure you add at least 2 glasses of unsweetened cranberry juice to your intake until the symptoms are gone.
- Always have a wee before and after sex.
- Make sure you empty your bladder properly when you wee. Once you've been, stand up and rock the pelvis back and forth and then sit down and see if you need to go again.
- Keep clean and dry and wear cotton pants.
- Shower daily and avoid perfumed soaps.
- Always wipe front to back to avoid bacteria entering the vagina.

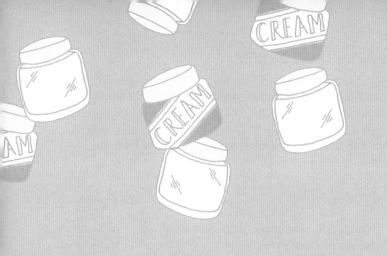

The Magical Middle

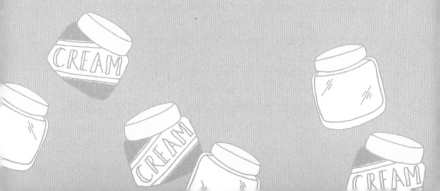

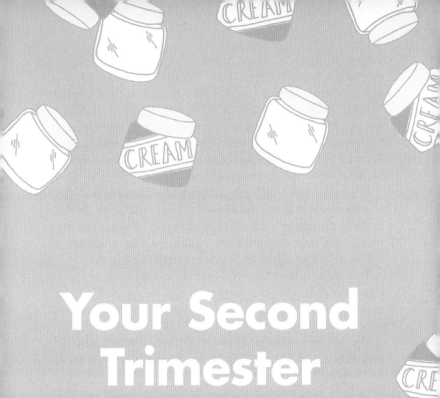

Your Second Trimester

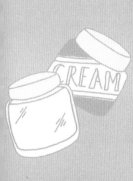
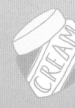
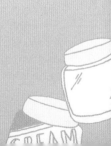

Before you know it, you've made it to the middle and things start to get really exciting! It can feel quite monumental as you transition from the first twelve weeks into the second trimester (weeks 12–28). If you have been feeling groggy and bone-tired so far, you may notice your energy begin to increase a little, resulting in you feeling a bit more like yourself again. Think of this time as the lull before the fiesta, when women often feel the most comfortable and well.

If, on the other hand, you continue to experience the weight of exhaustion and nausea throughout this next stage, do return to the first trimester section for our tips and advice, and be gentle with yourself. Reach out for support and remember all the incredible invisible work you are continuing to do.

Your body is very busy and your baby's development continues at an ever-speedy rate. Every day, your little bean continues to be more aware of the womb-dwelling world they inhabit.

You will also experience two of the most exciting parts of pregnancy. First, seeing your bump appear and grow, so that those around you start to notice the evidence that there is actually a tiny person in there. Your secret is finally out, and it can feel so liberating being able to talk openly about the highs and lows of pregnancy so far.

Secondly, starting to feel your baby's kicks and wiggles! You may be surprised at just how active your little human can be. It can be reassuring to start to see and feel their presence and become aware of their sleeping and active periods, and finally be able to put physical proof alongside that scan picture.

Pregnancy can be a time of feeling excited and joyous, but it can also have its challenges. Really nurturing, nourishing and caring for yourself and your growing babe continues to be very important and there are many ways that you can support your physical and mental wellbeing during your second trimester.

Remember to continue to follow your own instincts and intuition as to what you need during this time, and don't be surprised if the early nights are still calling you. It is important that you continue to check in on yourself and be aware of what you are feeling physically and mentally and make time to rest and recharge during this time.

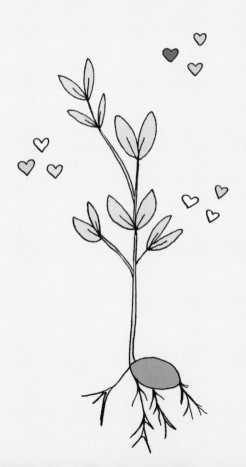

Caring for Your Changing Body

Hopefully, you'll find the second trimester affords you some time of feeling really well. Often (although by no means all the time for some women) the sickness and tiredness can dissipate, leaving you feeling rather energised compared to those early days. However, as your pregnancy progresses in this second trimester, your body will continue to change and adapt accordingly, making sure that the little one inside you has everything it needs to grow. It still blows us away that our bodies know how to do this all by themselves! That said, although there is no denying it is a joyous miracle, it can also feel like hard graft both emotionally and physically as your body works to care for you and your baby (or babies), leaving you feeling a little (or a lot) uncomfortable at times.

This is why we can't reiterate enough that self-care for mums-to-be is so important. Supporting yourself along the way with little hacks and treats here and there really will make the world of difference to how you feel physically and mentally as your journey continues.

Oh the aches!

You may start to feel more aches and pains than usual, partly due to baby growing and your bump becoming heavier to carry around, but mostly this is due to the wonderful hormone relaxin, which starts to increase through the second and third trimesters, to soften your body and prepare it for birth.

Softer ligaments may mean an increase in uncomfy sensations and twinges as our muscles strain a little under the pressure of supporting these extra-mobile joints! We talk a lot about supporting the pelvis through aches and pains on pages 49–51 but these tips below will also help support your ever-changing body through the second trimester.

- Epsom salt baths – there's nothing quite like a soak in the bath to ease tired, tense muscles – add some Epsom salts and you'll be in heaven! (See page 67 for all the benefits and instructions on usage.)

- Gentle exercise (see pages 37–38 for guidance) stretches muscles and increases blood circulation and lymphatic flow, which will allow muscles to be cleansed (flushing out toxins and lactic acid) and relaxed. Try to schedule in a regular time to get moving. The key here is little and often – 5 minutes a day is better than 1 hour a week!

- Don't forget to rest! Remember, your body is doing a lot of work quietly behind the scenes. You may not be able to see all the action, but you may certainly be feeling it some days – listen to your body and rest where possible when you feel the need.

- Bodywork – a trained bodywork therapist (who is qualified to work with pregnant women) can help work any tight muscles and support your body through its changes, helping limit the aches and pains you experience. Physiotherapy, osteopathy, remedial massage, reflexology and acupuncture are all wonderful supports to the pregnant body.

- Now is a good time to invest in a birthing ball if you haven't already got one. They are great for sitting on during pregnancy and birth and keeping baby nicely aligned.

Diastasis Rectus Abdominus (DRA)

There is little talk of DRA during pregnancy, but it becomes a big topic of conversation postnatally, especially when you want to return to exercise. DRA occurs when the tissues between the two sides of your abdominal muscles are stretched due to your growing baby, resulting in the feeling of there being a gap between them. This is often more obvious post-partum when there is no longer a stretch on the tissues.

Start these exercises in your second trimester to help gently stretch your abdominal muscles and improve your core muscle strength. You could even try and find a local pregnancy Pilates course to support you through your pregnancy and meet other mamas to be.

Cat-cow stretches with big belly breaths

1. Position yourself on your hands and knees, then let the weight of your belly drop down as you gently lift your head up and stick your bottom out.

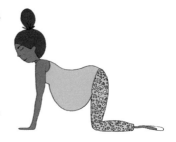

2. Take a deep breath in to allow the soft tissues across the front of your body to have a good stretch.

3. Reverse the movement, arch and round your back up like a cat and tuck your head and bottom underneath you as you breathe out. Repeat x 4.

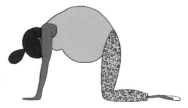

Tummy tucks

1. On all fours, with your back nice and flat, take a breath in and as you breathe out, try to tuck up the lower part of your tummy (bring your belly button towards your spine), while keeping your back and ribs still.

2. You will feel your bump being gently pulled up against gravity. Hold this for a few seconds, and then with an in-breath fully relax your tummy again.

Restless legs

Restless Legs Syndrome is a syndrome that causes unpleasant sensations in the legs, triggering the urge to move them. Some people feel it like a pulse in the legs, others like tight muscles with twitching. However yours plays out, it's no fun and can leave you feeling miserable and tired because it will disturb your sleep, sometimes keeping you awake. Try the following for relief from restless legs:

- Being deficient in magnesium and iron can make your symptoms worse, so ask your midwife to arrange a blood test to check your iron levels. You can also buy yourself a magnesium spray and spray it on the soles of your feet at night (it can be a bit prickly if you spray it directly onto your legs).

- Make sure that you have a few Epsom salt baths a week, as this is another good source of magnesium. It is important to use the right amount of Epsom salts – ideally 3 mugfuls in the bath – and soak for at least 20 minutes before bedtime (see page 67).

- Some gentle massage on the legs can help relax the muscles and alleviate symptoms.

- Walk around the house or garden for 10 minutes before bed to increase your circulation.

- Avoid caffeine.

- While sitting watching TV, alternate ice and heat on your legs. Use a cold pack and a hot water bottle and swap between the two every 5 minutes until symptoms lessen. Always make sure that you have a cover on the hot water bottle and ice pack to avoid burning the skin.

> **PLEASE NOTE:** Check with your midwife if you are having reoccurring calf pain accompanied by a red, hot area as this can be a sign of a blood clot. Although your risk factors for developing a deep vein thrombosis (DVT) are higher in pregnancy, it still only affects a small number of women, but will need urgent medical attention if it should happen.

Varicose veins and pesky piles

Increased blood flow and the extra weight from the pressure of your growing baby can cause veins below the uterus to become more stretched and swollen. This can result in haemorrhoids around or inside the anus and varicose veins on the legs or vulva. You can find out more about piles on pages 120–121, and about varicose veins in our vaginal health section, on page 54, however we highly recommend the following to help treat both problems:

- Epsom salt baths (see below for instructions)

- Putting your feet up to ease the pressure on both the rectum and the vulva.

- Use cold maternity pads to cool the tissue and reduce inflammation. See pages 120–121 for instructions on how to make these.

The mighty Epsom salts!

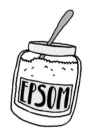

Epsom salts really are marvellous – a wonderful source of magnesium, they are useful in easing so many symptoms prenatally and also postnatally, including aches and pains, fluid retention and pelvic inflammation. We couldn't love them more! We would recommend ordering a big bag of them online, as you want to use a good amount. Don't buy hugely expensive stuff; good bath-grade Epsom salts is all you need, nothing fancy.

Pop three mugfuls in the bath, give it a good swirl to dissolve the salts and soak for at least 20 minutes before bed (you can feel a little woozy after a soak, so you'll probably sleep better too – win win!). Try adding a few drops of your favourite essential oils for a dose of extra luxury (see page 84), or some soothing chamomile tea to calm skin irritation (see page 56).

If your symptoms are bad, have a bath every other night and reduce as symptoms improve. If you have sensitive skin, or the salts make your skin itch, shower the salty water off quickly after the bath and you should be fine.

Pass the Gaviscon

Higher levels of progesterone, along with the pressure of the growing uterus on your stomach, can leave you with painful indigestion or acid reflux. Lots of mamas swear by Gaviscon, but there are also some great self-help tips that you can try to ease symptoms naturally.

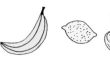

- Eat little and often so that you don't overload a squished tummy and sluggish digestive tract.

- Eat slowly and really chew your food so that your stomach has to do less work.

- Avoid spicy and greasy foods.

- Drink in between meals, not with your meal, to avoid diluting your stomach acid.

- Avoid eating right before bed, or laying down straight after food.

- Ginger, peppermint or chamomile tea are calming on the stomach.

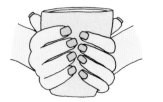

- Drink a mug of hot water with a slice of lemon first thing in the morning to kick-start your digestive system.

- Try coconut water, which is naturally soothing on the digestive tract.

- Almonds have an alkaline effect on the body — try eating a handful a day.

- Eat bananas, as these are very soothing on an acidic digestive tract.

- Chew sugar-free gum after meals (not in between) — this produces additional saliva and keeps the stomach acid from rising in the oesophagus.

- If it's making it hard to sleep, try sitting up in bed propped up with a few pillows.

Project Intuition!

Over the years of working with expectant mums, we have lost count of the number of times women have told us they were worried about going to see their midwife or doctor for fear that they would be 'wasting their time'. Believe us when we say: if you feel out of sorts and your instinct is telling you that you do not feel right, or that the changes you are experiencing are not as you would expect, then we would much rather you were seen by your local health professionals than sit at home worrying. If it is found you are having any atypical changes or symptoms, then you can access the care you need. Alternatively, if you and baby are found to be well and no further support is needed at this time, then you can rest easy with a little more knowledge about what you are experiencing and a spoonful of reassurance that everything is going as expected.

Always remember that you know yourself better than anyone! You are your own expert and the very best person to notice when you physically feel off-kilter. We have learned to really trust the instinct of a mother (or mother-to-be) throughout pregnancy and birth, so we know how to care for her in the best way possible. Remember: 'If in doubt, get checked out.'

It is SO easy to type any pregnancy sensation you may be experiencing into a search engine and frighten yourself silly with all the unqualified suggestions thrown back your way. Instead, phone your antenatal ward (a phone number should be on your maternity notes) and book in to be seen asap OR, if you feel it can wait, write it on a sticky note and pop it on your maternity papers to remind yourself to mention it at your next midwife appointment.

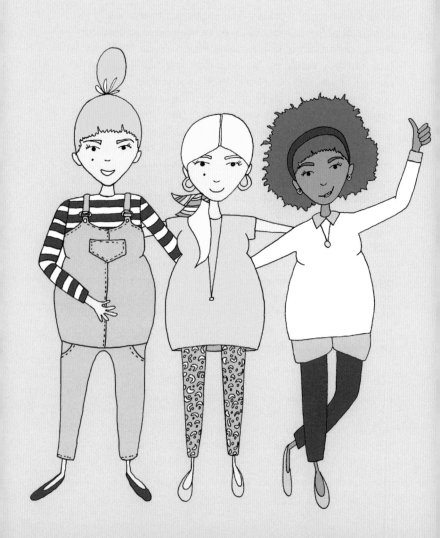

Building a Tribe

It really is important to put some time aside now to consider who and what will enrich your experience during pregnancy, labour and the postnatal period. Do a bit of research and look into where you can find professionals and other mums locally who can become your self-selected tribe, enhancing your experience of growing and birthing a baby and becoming a new mother. We are very lucky these days that there are so many choices available, and more ways than ever to reach out and find exactly what it is that you are looking for, whether it be antenatal, hypnobirthing or pregnancy yoga classes or just simply creating a new network of mum-to-be friends who can go through this journey with you, in real time. Whether it be your first or fourth baby, it's still so lovely to have that knowing smile or words of encouragement from another mother, who has been experiencing the same aches and pains, name-choosing dilemmas and pregnancy insomnia as you.

Pregnancy and birth team

We have seen it all: supporting mums coming into hospital alone, with just their partner or maybe also a mum, sister or friend to offer another layer of TLC. We have also seen women bring a complete entourage in, although it is worth noting that many units cap the amount of birth partners you can have in a hospital or a birth centre at 2 or 3, for security and safety reasons. However, if you're planning a home birth then you can have as few or as many of your nearest and dearest as you like!

It is increasingly popular to hire a doula for added help, knowledge and guidance, before, during and/or after the birth. This can be especially useful if you do not have family or friends nearby and feel you would benefit from a familiar face to support you. If you are toying with the idea of hiring either an independent midwife or doula for some or all of your pregnancy and birth, it is worth meeting and booking them early (in your second trimester). Places are often limited, as in order for them to be present and readily available to the women they care for, they usually only take on a few clients.

Solo mums

Whether you have planned to go through it yourself or have found yourself unexpectedly taking on your pregnancy journey solo, there are some brilliant ways to top up your mum gang and make sure you don't feel like you're in this alone. It's a little bit like the first day of school: everyone is in the same boat, going through this brilliant, challenging and enriching change in their lives, so conversations are freely opened. Once your pregnancy is visible, common ground is obvious and often easy to build upon!

Our top tips to build your community of mum chums

- Join an antenatal class/birth preparation/hypnobirthing or fourth trimester class and get to meet other expectant mums. If this is not your first baby, there may be a good refresher session held locally that means you can meet other mums who are pregnant again. It can be great for your partner too, and gives them an opportunity to get involved in the preparation and parenthood community.

- Find a pregnancy fitness class or yoga group that will mean you get to see the same mums-to-be regularly and build up some new friendships before your babies arrive. If you feel like the group gels well, suggest a regular meet-up when your maternity leave begins and get that tea and cake group started!

- Get hooked up! It's likely that friends of yours will know someone else locally who is due at a similar time to you. See if they can share your details, arrange a natter over coffee and see where that takes you.

- Tap into social media groups. We know they get a bad rep sometimes, but there are some good online communities. Although getting outside is important, it can be reassuring to know you can reach out and chat with other parents, even on the days when you don't leave the house and find yourself under a snoozing baby for long periods of time! You may also find online mums turn into pals who you meet up with face-to-face on the regular.

- Try using a mummy-meet-up app to find out if there are any events going on near you. This is a great way to connect with other parents in the area. If you have other children, you may also find other parents-to-be that need to occupy a busy toddler like you.

- Depending on how much time you have, you could look at helping out at a playgroup or children's 'quality seconds' jumble sale, which are often put on for local mums by antenatal groups. You can meet other parents and nab a bargain in that pile of pre-loved baby garb!

- If you are growing more than one baby, you may wish to attend a local twin/triplets group or workshop and gain some tips from other multiple mamas.

Positive vibes only, please!

We really encourage the mamas we work with to surround themselves with the right sort of birth tales when it comes to fuelling their beliefs and imagination as they prepare for their own experience. It's important to notice if there is a family member, friend or even colleague, who keeps sharing scary birthing stories with you. You are NOT the outlet for their fears and worries, and it is completely inappropriate for them to voice these stories with you as you approach the birth of your own baby.

When you are trying to approach birth, feeling calm and in control of your adrenaline and promoting your birthing hormones, namely oxytocin and endorphins (see pages 178–179 for more on these magic hormones), such information can be detrimental to your birthing mind and body. We are not saying that you should expect birth to be 'perfect', whatever that might mean to you, but we are encouraging you to know that however birth plays out, you can have the right people around you and go into your experience with positivity. If you find that people are relaying terrible tales to you, there has to be a moment when you raise up your hand, stop them in their tracks and remind them that this might not be the best time to be telling you this. We are not trying to disregard another person's experience, but there really is a time and a place.

No comparison

For some reason, pregnancy and new motherhood can make women compare themselves to others and worry that they are not doing it all well enough. It's probably because we are even more sensitive than usual, making sure we are preparing for everything that our baby will need. There is no right or wrong, and you're only human and can't do everything! You are doing the best you can, as is everyone else, and that, my friend, is absolutely enough. Your tribe needs to be there to help lift your spirits and give you that knowing smile and fist pump when you feel like you need some extra encouragement.

As time goes on, your confidence will grow and you will soon discover what works for your family, and that is the most important thing. So acknowledge that it's very normal to compare yourself to others occasionally and then remind yourself what a super job you are doing and how you will be the best mama your baby could wish for!

We recommend writing down a list of all the amazing things you have done so far and that you plan to do as pregnancy progresses for you and your baby – from taking vitamins and attending appointments and scans to cutting down on certain foods and drinks you love. You are likely to see that you are doing the best you can and that that is all you can ask of yourself.

Nourishing Grub: Part 2

Hopefully, if it hasn't already, then very soon the sickness or tiredness will be starting to lift (at least a bit) and you will be feeling up for cooking and eating heartier meals again. The second trimester can be a lovely time to eat well and enjoy nourishing yourself, so we've included a couple of easy one-pot recipes, along with simple, nutritious breakfast and lunch ideas.

Quinoa Porridge

A filling healthy breakfast that is gluten-free and easy to digest. You can use oats instead of quinoa if you prefer – note that they will cook more quickly and require less milk.

Serves 1

1 mug of quinoa
400ml drinking coconut milk
½ mug of water
3 tablespoons maple syrup
1 teaspoon vanilla extract
¼ teaspoon salt

Place all the ingredients in a saucepan and bring to the boil.

Reduce the heat and simmer, stirring often, for 20–30 minutes until cooked. Add extra water or milk if needed.

Once cooked, add some toppings to your porridge to bring it to life. We like:

- Chopped pear, pecans and flaked coconut
- Honey, walnuts and chopped plums
- Grated apple, chopped dates and ground cinnamon
- Chopped banana, chia seeds and peanut butter

Bone Broth Noodles

Bone broth is SO full of goodness and is such a good tonic. Drink it on its own or use it as the perfect base to any soup or stew. Make a big stock of broth, then keep a batch in the fridge for a week and freeze the rest. The broth will last up to six months in the freezer.

Makes 1.5 litres

1 x chicken carcass from a roast chicken (or a pack of chicken wings if you don't have a carcass)
1 tablespoon apple cider vinegar
1 carrot, roughly chopped
1 onion, peeled and roughly chopped
1 celery stick, roughly chopped
2 bay leaves
a few peppercorns
1 teaspoon sea salt

Place the chicken carcass in a large pan or slow cooker. Add the apple cider vinegar, chopped veg, bay leaves, pepper and salt. Cover with cold water and bring to the boil. Reduce the heat and simmer very gently for 6–8 hours, skimming occasionally to remove any froth and topping up the water as required. Once cooked, strain the broth and store in heatproof containers, bottles or jars. Before you use the broth, scrape off any fatty layer that may have formed.

Note: If time doesn't allow, you can cheat and buy good-quality bone broth from the supermarket and use for the noodle soup below.

Bone broth noodle soup
Warm up a batch of your homemade bone broth in a pan. Allow about 300ml per person.

Add some chopped carrots and shredded cabbage. Bring to the boil and simmer for 15–20 minutes, until the veg is tender.

Add some dried noodles, and some cooked chicken, chopped spring onions and peas and simmer for 5 minutes until cooked. Serve immediately, with crusty bread.

One-pot Veg and Lentil Casserole ....

Super-quick and easy – perfect for chucking in the oven and popping your feet up while it cooks! This is a lovely nourishing and warming way of getting your five-a-day! And it's full of iron.

Serves 4

1 onion, peeled and roughly chopped
225g Puy or green lentils
1 bay leaf
1 litre vegetable stock or your bone broth from page 77
2 leeks, trimmed, washed and sliced
2 potatoes, peeled and chopped
2 carrots, peeled and chopped
3 courgettes, chopped
1 celery stick, chopped
1 red pepper, halved, deseeded and chopped
1 tablespoon lemon juice
salt and pepper
crusty bread and/or a green salad, to serve

Preheat the oven to 180°C/160°F fan.

Add the onion, lentils and bay leaf to a large casserole dish.

Pour over the stock, cover and cook in the oven for 1 hour.

Add the rest of the veg, stir thoroughly and season with salt and pepper. Cover and cook in the oven for another hour.

Remove from the oven, discard the bay leaf and stir in the lemon juice. Serve immediately with some nice crusty bread and/or a green salad.

Variation: Pimp up your casserole with some cooked chicken or cooked chopped sausage for a meaty alternative.

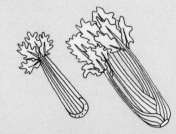

mocktails

Just remember: no boozing doesn't have to mean no fun. Rustle up one of these tasty cocktails next time you fancy a tipple.

Each mocktail serves 1.

Maple Mojito

10 fresh mint leaves
1 lime, quartered
a glug of maple syrup
ice cubes and soda water,
  to serve

Crush the mint leaves a little to release their flavour, then place in the bottom of a glass.

Squeeze the juice from the lime quarters into the glass then drop the lime pieces in.

Pour over a glug of maple syrup, add ice cubes and top with soda water.

Mango Mule

2 slices of cucumber
1 tablespoon honey
50ml mango juice
50ml fresh lime juice
ice cubes
150ml ginger beer

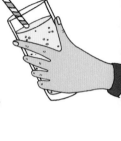

Crush the cucumber and honey at the bottom of a cocktail shaker with the end of a wooden spoon.

Add the mango juice, lime juice and some ice cubes and shake vigorously for 10 seconds.

Strain into a glass and top up with the ginger beer. Stir and serve.

How to Get More ZZZs

Unfortunately, many women find that their sleep becomes disturbed during pregnancy. Hormonal changes, sore hips from side sleeping, a nocturnal wriggly baby, restless legs or an over-sensitive bladder – to name a few causes – are not very conducive to a good night's sleep. Let's look at all the little tips and tricks we can use to get better kip!

Get a good bedtime routine

- Don't eat too late. Your digestion is slower during pregnancy and you're more likely to suffer with heartburn. Eat little and often, and avoid too much fat, sugars or carbs before bed.

- Avoid screen time an hour before bed. Read a relaxing book, listen to the radio, a podcast or your hypnobirthing downloads, or write in a journal instead.

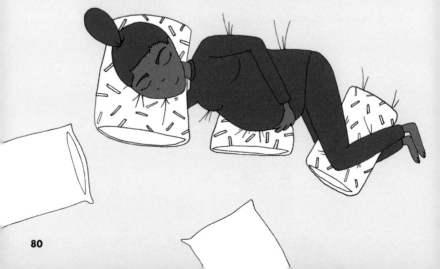

- Wash the day away with a bath or shower. Not only will this relax muscles, but it will also help clear your mind.

- Wear your cosiest garb. Pregnancy is not a fashion show. Think snug, loose-fitting, elasticated and soft. This will help send the signal of relaxation to your body.

- Turn the lights down low. Light hinders the secretion of melatonin so keeping the lights off or down low really does help us to sleep better. If you prefer total darkness try using a sleep mask or blackout blinds. Lie comfortably in the low lighting and focus on your breath – encouraging a longer out-breath than in-breath. Try visualising breathing around the sides of a rectangle: in-breath around the short side, and out-breath along the long side.

All the pillows
Whether you buy a fancy pregnancy pillow or just bolster yourself up with some more bed pillows, you will definitely need some extra cushioning to sleep comfortably and to support your body in the right way. THE most important thing you can do to help you to sleep in a side position more comfortably, while at the same time protecting your hips and pelvis from strain and discomfort, is to sleep with enough pillows between your knees.

What we are aiming for is for your knee to be in line with your hip. If your knee is dipping down, you will be hanging off the hip and gluteal muscles, meaning they will stay fired up and working all night when they could be resting. This positioning can also create a pull on the lumbar back, resulting in soreness. Investing in a good-quality soft mattress topper can help by cushioning the hips while sleeping in a side position.

Turning over the right way!

Let's face it, turning over with a baby on board isn't easy! But side sleeping means we often have to turn regularly to avoid achy hips. Flinging yourself over using your leg to propel you from one side to the other can really twang the muscles in your groin and lower back, and this can result in inflammation and leave you aching. If you are suffering from any pain or instability in the pelvis such as Pelvic Girdle Pain (PGP) you definitely need to try the technique below!

Kneesy does it
A much better way to turn over at night, and one
that certainly puts much less strain on your pelvis,
is to first roll onto your hands and knees. So, if you
are lying on your left side, roll over to the left and
gently manoeuvre onto your hands and knees.
Then, shuffle over onto your right side. This way
you can swap sides without putting any strain on
the pelvis at all.

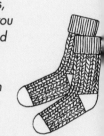

Keep it cool

Being too hot can interfere with good sleep. In the summertime, leave windows open if possible, leave blinds or curtains shut during the day and try using a fan (pointing away from you directly, but circulating the air). Try having a cool shower before bed, use cotton sheets and wear minimal clothes. On a really hot, clammy night you could use a refreshing cool flannel over your body, on the back of the neck, the forehead or under your breasts to help cool you down. And try popping your pillowcase in the freezer in a sealable bag for 10 minutes before bedtime – once it's back on your pillow it will feel lovely and cool.

Restless legs

Restless legs are a pain – literally. We have outlined lots of ways to ease the symptoms of this condition earlier, on pages 65–66, but Epsom salt baths and a good old leg rub are our firm favourites.

Crazy dreams

Dreams can feel more vivid during pregnancy due to the hormone changes in our body, and also underlying anxieties can often play out when we sleep.

If a dream proves particularly upsetting or alarming, try writing it down to get it out of your head before going back to sleep. Look at it in the daytime to see if there may be an unexplored worry you could do some work on releasing.

Wee-athon!

With little one wriggling around and putting pressure on your bladder it is no surprise we can often wake up in the night needing a wee. There isn't much we can do about this, but do try limiting your water intake an hour or two before bedtime if it's really bothering you, and also make sure that you empty your bladder fully when you go – see page 57.

If you do wake up in the night needing a wee, try and keep the lighting low, so you don't disturb yourself too much and you can get back to sleep easily.

Night-time snack

A hungry tummy does not help us to fall back to sleep, so try taking a flask of herbal tea and a pack of biscuits or oatcakes to bed to settle any night-time hunger pangs.

Naps – so good, it should be illegal not to!

If your sleep is disturbed night after night, then do try to catch up a bit with a daytime nap. Mid-morning or straight after lunch are fab times to take one, no later though or else it can turn into a danger nap and may disturb your night-time sleep.

Herbs and oils

Herbal teas such as valerian and chamomile can be wonderful to aid a restful night's sleep.

Essential oils can also soothe and settle the mind and body. Try using 4 drops of your favourite oil in a diffuser or place 4 drops on a piece of tissue and rest it on your bedside table or pillow so you can gently breathe in the lovely rest-inducing pong. You can also add 6 drops of essential oil to 2ml carrier oil and add it to your bath: pour the mixture into the running water, as this will help the oil blend into the bath water.

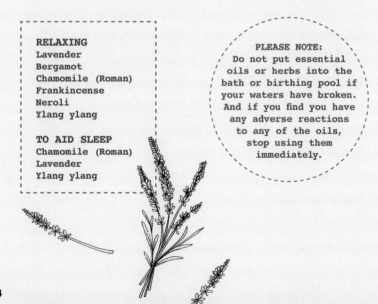

RELAXING
Lavender
Bergamot
Chamomile (Roman)
Frankincense
Neroli
Ylang ylang

TO AID SLEEP
Chamomile (Roman)
Lavender
Ylang ylang

PLEASE NOTE:
Do not put essential oils or herbs into the bath or birthing pool if your waters have broken. And if you find you have any adverse reactions to any of the oils, stop using them immediately.

Placenta Encapsulation

If you are planning to have your placenta encapsulated, you will need to book that in during your second or early third trimester. The practitioner will then give you a kit to keep the placenta sterile once you have birthed it, and if you are staying in hospital overnight, the hospital will keep it in the fridge for you. Once baby is born, let the placenta specialist know and they will come and collect it at a mutually convenient time and take it away to prepare your pills.

It is suggested that dehydrating the placenta and preparing it into tablets for mum to take can help with:

- A release of CRH – a stress-releasing hormone
- Low mood
- Increasing milk production
- Replenishing depleted iron levels
- Increasing energy levels

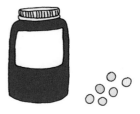

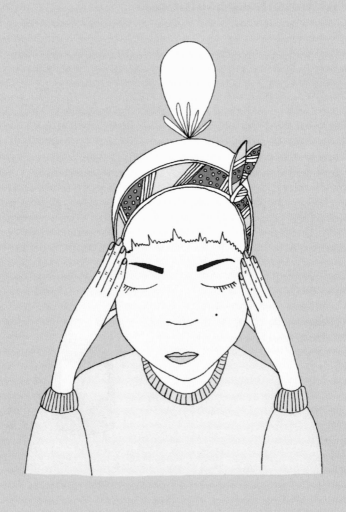

Minding a Mum-to-be

Pregnancy is an incredible period of growth and change for a woman, both physically and mentally. It is a different experience for everyone and where some women will feel gorgeous and glowing, and fall in love with that growing bump, others can feel unsexy, exhausted and nervous about the physical changes and what parenthood will bring.

Despite the truly fascinating and miraculous work your body is doing in order to grow an actual human being from scratch, we understand that this identity shift can feel challenging and there is no shame in admitting that the physical changes and pregnancy-related symptoms can take some adjusting to.

The truth is there is no right or wrong way to feel about pregnancy and it is definitely okay not to enjoy every moment. That does not make you ungrateful; it's just a reflection of the fact that pregnancy can be tough at times. It is important to cut yourself some slack and be kind to yourself, as your mind, body and identity go through some pretty significant transformations.

As the weeks go on you may find that you start to find wonder in that growing bump, especially once you start to look pregnant and your partner, friends and family can share their excitement with you as your baby belly (soon to be littlest love) starts to show itself off to the world. Read on to the next section, though, for more information on how to recognise when things aren't quite right.

Perinatal mental health

Every one of us has both mental health and physical health. Some women will find they feel really mentally well during pregnancy and on the whole find the experience joyful and positive. However, others may notice uncomfortable and challenging alterations in their mood, thoughts and feelings.

You may have noticed that antenatal mental health illnesses get far less air-time than postnatal depression (PND), yet with a significant number of women suffering from compromised mental wellbeing in pregnancy, it is about time we started sharing more knowledge and raising awareness on the matter.

Perinatal mental health conditions can follow on from pre-existing conditions or creep out of nowhere. They are illnesses and not a reflection of you as a woman or as a mother-to-be. Depression and anxiety that starts in pregnancy can often be related to hormonal and chemical changes happening within the brain, invisible from the outside.

If you start to notice some changes in your mood, it can be very helpful to keep a mood diary. Be curious about the thoughts you are having (especially if they are out of character) and note the way you are feeling physically in response. And do remember you can always talk to your midwife about any concerns.

Bump anxiety

If there is one thing that we hear about time and again, it's women feeling like they become public property when they are expecting. The personal comments and uninvited touching can feel intrusive and overly familiar, galloping over boundaries that would not normally be crossed. Flippant comments, in particular, are a bug-bear of ours. It's like everyone has an opinion on what your bump should or shouldn't look like. Recently, we were working with a lady who had convinced herself that she had gestational diabetes because of all the comments she had received about her 'big' bump, and then right in front of us someone approached her, put their hand on her tummy (uninvited) and chortled, 'how many weeks to go lovely? Are you sure it's not twins?' Just to clarify, she was thirty weeks pregnant with baby number three and was measuring well within normal limits, and yet the comments still came, resulting in some serious bump anxiety.

The fact is that bumps (just like bodies) come in all different shapes and sizes. Some women naturally carry lower, some wider, some in a neat little ball, some barely noticeable and others taking up every single bit of space, with their bump popping out from early on! From around twenty-four weeks your midwife will start measuring your bump and if they feel that they would like more information regarding your baby's size, they will organise a scan for you.

We know it is easier said than done, but try to ignore people's silly and thoughtless comments where possible. If it is someone you see regularly, maybe let them know that those seemingly harmless remarks are actually making you worry, so could they just STOP...thank you!

WRITE A MOOD DIARY

- Carry a notebook around with you and take brief notes throughout the day regarding your thoughts and feelings. Jot down how you feel in your mood, such as edgy, nervous, low or vacant. Take note if there are any triggers that seem to make you feel worse, such as poor sleep, overwhelming workload or watching or hearing an unsettling story.

- Record if you are noticing any uncomfortable and unwelcome physical sensations alongside a low or anxious mood, such as a tight chest, dizziness, racing heart or tingly arms and legs.

- Be aware if you see any changes in your behaviour in response to these feelings, such as not wanting to leave the house and avoiding friends and family, or avoiding busy places, or perhaps needing to be in the company of others constantly as you have started finding it unnerving to be alone.

If you notice that what you are experiencing is affecting your day-to-day life, we strongly suggest talking to your nearest and dearest about how you are feeling. We really do believe that a problem shared is a problem halved, and by acknowledging and opening up about what we are going through, we may disempower these scary thoughts and feelings, stop self-blaming and regain a sense of control in the healing process. There are also many options available through your midwife and GP, such as support with gentle mind and body exercises and mindfulness tools, and talking therapies including cognitive behavioural therapy (CBT) that can help you change the way you think and behave. There are also various medication options that can be utilised to help you feel well again.

It is important to ensure all women are given the best chance of fast recovery from perinatal mental health difficulties, as we all deserve the right to experience those moments of joy as we approach motherhood.

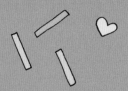

"

'Around week twenty-four I started to lose myself. At first, I couldn't put my finger on why I was feeling so flat and disconnected to my pregnancy. I couldn't sleep and felt constantly sick with worry. After experiencing some intrusive thoughts, I decided I needed to reach out for support and spoke to my midwife. I was referred to see a mental health specialist and was diagnosed with antenatal depression and anxiety.

My four-year-old son overheard a conversation I was having with my husband and asked me why I was going to see the doctor, to which I answered, "Mummy has a poorly head, but I'm going to get better." And I did just that. Through CBT, mindfulness and a low dose of anxiety meds I started sleeping again and made a full recovery by the time my second beautiful boy arrived.'

TORI, MUM OF TWO

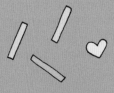

It's All About the Calm

Whether you are feeling openly worried or calm as a cucumber about your pregnancy or the birth itself, we highly recommend using the following tools to help soothe any anxieties that may be bubbling away – or to set yourself up with ways to help manage such feelings that could crop up later on. These techniques can also start preparing you for birth. It may seem a bit early, but in our experience incorporating ways to care for your mind and reduce adrenaline and stress hormones early on can be extremely helpful and empowering. It can have a positive effect for an expectant mum at any stage of her baby-growing journey!

Simple practical techniques, such as positive affirmations, visualisations and relaxation scripts prove to be useful over and over again and the great news is they won't cost you a thing! Practise these regularly so they become second nature to you and you can call on them when you need them.

Pregnancy brain re-org

Incredible fact alert! Your brain has the ability to go through a significant re-organisation, known as neuroplasticity, at certain key points in your lifetime, including pregnancy. During this life event, the brain actually changes shape and redirects some of the blood flow away from short-term memory (aha, that's what causes 'baby brain'!) and to the parts of the brain that are in control of empathy and responding to sensory stimulation. Therefore, when your baby arrives, you will be able to recognise when they need you and will be driven to respond to them swiftly. It is a very clever evolutionary development. However, it's worth knowing that it can leave you feeling a little more reactive to outside sensory stimulation during pregnancy, as your brain primes your motherly protective mode. Have you noticed that loud noises, busy places and bright lights can make you feel a little more edgy than they used to? That could well be your brain just encouraging you to be more vigilant to your surroundings, like a bird on their nest, guarding their precious egg. Tap into the adrenaline-relieving techniques mentioned throughout this book – such as breathing exercises, stretching and massage techniques – whenever you feel that you could benefit from soothing these reactive sensations.

Hypnobirthing

When it comes to keeping calm and in control about pregnancy and birth, many women find hypnobirthing very helpful. In essence, hypnobirthing is another form of antenatal education that places more emphasis on how your mind, hormones and birthing body work together, giving you simple and practical ways to keep calm, no matter how your birth unfolds. It's really not as kooky as it may sound, and is actually based on the science of optimising the birthing hormones and calming fears and concerns about birth that may be holding us back and leading to feelings of loss of control and intense discomfort.

In short, fear + tension = pain

Hypnobirthing recognises how the mind and body work together like a continuous feedback mechanism, sending internal messages back and forth within the birthing body. When fear is present, we can trigger adrenaline quickly because we are responding to what is happening to us with a very primal and reactive part of our brain. It's all about learning and practising simple ways to manage and lower adrenaline and encourage oxytocin and endorphins to thrive.

To make it as easy as possible to get on board the positivity train, we have included a lovely, uplifting and confidence-boosting list of affirmations, and a partner relaxation script on pages 126–129 that you can use to encourage that all-important positive and confident mindset!

You can also find lots of relaxing and fear-releasing hypnobirthing tracks and MP3s online and available to download. Practising using relaxation scripts, breathwork (see pages 130–135), massage and the daily use of powerful and positive pregnancy and birth affirmations during pregnancy gives you the best chance of feeling calm and in control as you approach your baby's birth.

Affirmations

Using positive affirmations regularly during pregnancy can help turn around any self-sabotaging inner dialogue you may be experiencing. It's not uncommon to focus on the scary stories that we have heard throughout the years and forget that pregnancy and birth can be positive and empowering experiences. We want to share with you our favourite affirmations and highly recommend you write up the ones that speak to you, plus any others you think of yourself, and put them up around your home in places you (and your partner) will see regularly. Pop one on the toilet door, by the kettle and by your bed so that reading them becomes a part of your normal day-to-day routine. Later on you can also make them a part of your birth bag by writing them up on a paper chain of bunting or pieces of paper and sticking them up on the wall wherever you plan to birth.

affirmations

Make time to focus on the following:

- I make time every day to connect with my baby

- I look forward to the birth of my baby

- My partner is with me every step of our journey

- I can encourage my oxytocin and endorphins to thrive

- My baby and I are surrounded by love and support

- I feel calm and in control

- Every day I am one step closer to seeing your little face

- I trust and celebrate my body

- My baby and my body are designed to work together

- I can respond with calm confidence, however birth unfolds

- I am in the right place, with the right people supporting me

- We are open and ready for whatever birth we experience

- My body is strong and powerful

- Thousands of other women are birthing across the world, at the same time as me

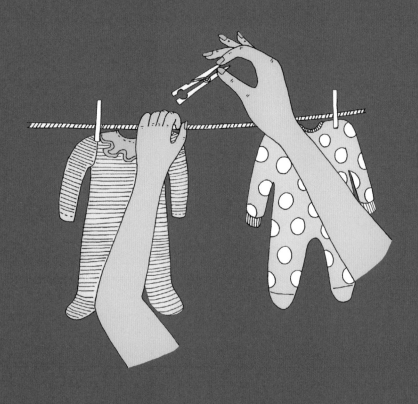

Connecting With Your Baby

For many women, the idea that there is actually a human being inside that bump seems so bizarre. A tiny little person made by you, developing and growing during every single moment of your pregnancy. Some women absolutely love the feeling of their changing and expanding body as their baby grows and know that they will really miss their wiggling bump once the baby arrives. Others find pregnancy to be a means to an end, with the arrival of the baby being the target. There is no right or wrong way to experience this baby-making lark. However you are feeling, we have put together a list of some lovely ways you can pay homage to the incredible work your body is doing and start to build a sweet connection with your little one before they arrive. See over the page for our bump-bonding ideas.

BUMP BONDING

TALK, READ AND SING TO YOUR BUMP

Did you know your baby can hear sounds from as early as eighteen weeks?! By the time they get to twenty-four weeks they are able to tune in to sounds inside and outside the womb. It's well known that when a baby is born, they respond positively to familiar sounds, especially mums, dads, close friends and family that have been around a lot during the pregnancy, and even the music that you listen to. Tap into that opportunity to connect with them through talking and singing to them. (Fact: they don't care if you're tone deaf; they will love your voice regardless.)

TICKLE CHASE

Babies are tactile little beings. We know from scans that they enjoy sucking their thumbs and fingers and playing with their cord. During a busy day it's not always easy to notice every movement, but when you are home, take time to really tune in to the wiggles. Stroke them back, and gently nudge their poking foot or hand in return.

DANCE WITH YOUR BABY

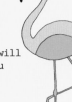

Babies are soothed by movement. That doesn't mean you have to be active constantly, but without realising it, you will be swaying them back and forth throughout your pregnancy. We can see their response to movement once they are born, because they often settle well when we move or jiggle them gently in our arms. Play some music, wrap your arms around that glorious belly and move to the beat.

BRING YOUR BREATH TO YOUR BABY

As you know, we highly recommend you practise breathing techniques throughout pregnancy to help stay calm and to prepare you for using breathwork in labour. Simple techniques, such as 3 Flamingos (see page 26), can soothe and calm you, and in turn, your baby will be soothed too.

MAKE A MEMORY BOX

Start a box of the special items that will have meaning for you and your baby. That could be congratulations cards, bump photos, a letter you've written to your baby, even the positive pregnancy test (yep, we kept ours). When the baby arrives, keep adding to it with their hospital tags, first outfit, cord clamp, celebratory messages and anything else that might be important to you as the years go on.

SPEND TIME IN THEIR SPACE

One of the exciting things that makes the arrival of your baby feel more real is preparing and holding their tiny things. Whatever sweet corner you have prepared for your baby, spend some time thinking about them being in that space when they arrive. You may have bought a special picture for the wall, have been given a cosy blankie, or have their babygros folded neatly waiting for them. Whatever you have done in preparation, sit in that space and give your bump a cuddle. It won't be long until they are here making use of that carefully planned nook.

LOOK AT THEIR SCAN PICTURE

You're probably wondering who in the world this little person will be? Carry your scan pic with you and take a peek to connect with your baby. We know that if a new mum is parted from their infant and wants to express milk, looking at a photo can give them a rush of oxytocin which can help their milk to flow. That little scan picture may help encourage some pre-birth bonding.

KEEP A PREGNANCY JOURNAL

Even though it feels at times like pregnancy will never end, it does. When it's over and you transition into the postnatal period, your memories will start to fade a little. Parenthood can feel like a whirlwind, so it can be lovely to document the journey. Even if you aren't feeling in awe of your pregnant body right now, take some photos to look back; you will be surprised how quickly you forget what it felt like to have that beautiful bump.

GET YOUR PARTNER ON BOARD

Aside from the antenatal and hypnobirthing classes, there are day-to-day ways to get your partner bonding with baby. Spend time getting them to gently nudge and feel the kicks and wiggles. This will also help you feel connected with your partner on the road to parenthood.

Self-massage and Partner Massage

There are so many benefits to having regular massages during pregnancy – it can help ease aches and pains, and provide some much-needed 'time out' for mum-to-be to enjoy bonding with her expanding bump. All that growing a baby is tiring! A bit of TLC can do you the world of good. Massage will also often result in a fantastic night's sleep afterwards, as the body is put back in balance, and this can be very welcome, especially later on in your pregnancy when sleep patterns can become a bit more erratic.

If time or finances don't allow a trip to a professional, don't worry! We've included a few sections in this book (see the following pages and pages 136–137 and 182–183) that teach you easy massages that you can do on yourself, massages that you could ask a partner, friend or family member to do for you, and a couple of stretches which will really relax those muscles and keep your wonderful body working well.

PLEASE NOTE: Only massage on the muscle, never on bone, as this is very sensitive and can be painful. Do not massage over open wounds. Do not massage if mum-to-be is feeling unwell or has a temperature. Do not massage on an empty tummy otherwise you can feel lightheaded; or on a full tummy, or you may be uncomfortable. Please avoid massaging too deeply into the middle of the tops of the shoulders and the inside of the ankles, where there are some acupressure points that can stimulate labour.

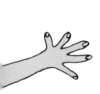

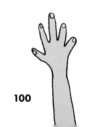

Butt & Ball

This self-massage is a really great way to release the bum and hip muscles that are working hard to keep your pelvis stable, and which can also be a bit achy from sleeping on your side.

1. Grab a trusty tennis ball and sandwich it between your bottom and the wall.

2. Use your weight to press in against the ball until you feel it affect the muscle.

3. Now move left to right, or up and down, to roll the ball over the bum muscles.

4. When you feel a tender spot stop there and press in a little more until you feel the muscle relax.

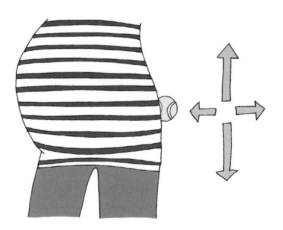

Seated back massage

Those back muscles are working hard to support the weight of your growing bump, counterbalancing the change in your centre of gravity and helping to stabilise looser joints. There's no avoiding a bit of back strain in pregnancy, but a good back massage once a week (more, if your partner is willing) will make all the difference in easing those aches and pains!

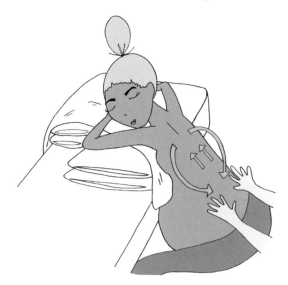

Instructions for your partner:

1. Sit mum-to-be on a stool at the kitchen table. Place some pillows on the table so that she can rest against them. If you don't have a stool, use a normal dining chair, but get her to sit on it sideways, so that her back is clear and the back of the chair is to the side.

2. Sit behind your partner and, using some nut-free oil such as grapeseed or coconut oil, start to massage her back, helping to relax the muscles that are working hard to support her growing bump.

3. Starting at the bottom of the back, place your hands either side of her spine.

4. Glide the hands up towards her head, stroke over the tops of the shoulders and then stroke the hands down her sides, finally bringing them back into their starting position at either side of the spine.

5. Repeat as many times as she likes! This is a really calming and relaxing massage for body and mind.

   Note: The slower you massage, the more calming the effect on her will be.

Bonding belly massage

Get your birth partner to give you a lovely gentle belly massage. This is not only great to support the expanding muscles, but baby loves it too and usually responds with a lovely little wriggle for you, so this can be a nice way for you and your birth partner to bond with baby.

Laying on your side with a pillow between your knees, your massage partner can then stand or kneel behind you, so that they can comfortably reach over your bump.

Instructions for your partner:

1. Place your hand on the centre of her bump, over the belly button. Get her to take a few big breaths, feeling her tummy expanding into your hand to relax.

2. Now, using a little nut-free oil, glide both hands gently and slowly over her tummy in a clockwise motion. Keep making clockwise circles with both hands, bringing one hand up off the bump to cross over when needed.

3. Now, place one hand on the tummy and one on the lower back and gently massage in a clockwise circle, with both hands mirroring each other. Continue to massage for a few minutes or until she has had enough!

   Note: It is important to only work in a clockwise motion on the abdomen so that you are following the natural flow of the digestive system.

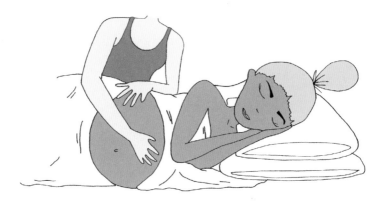

The chest opener stretch

This is such a great stretch to open the chest, stretch into the ribs and wake up and relax the shoulder muscles.

1. Start by kneeling on the floor with the tops of your feet pressed against the floor and either a yoga mat or cushion under your knees.

2. Sit back on your heels, round your shoulders, drop your head and let your arms hang down to the front of your body to stretch the backs of the shoulders.

3. Squeeze your bottom muscles and inhale as you come up to high kneeling, lifting your gaze up to the sky, stretching your arms up and out to the side and feeling your chest opening.

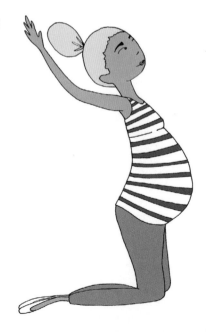

4. As you exhale, come back to your heels, dropping the arms to the front of the body, dropping your head, chin to chest, and rounding your shoulders to feel the stretch on the back.

5. Repeat 4 times.

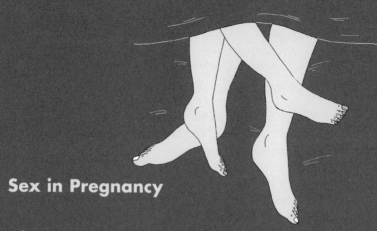

Sex in Pregnancy

When it comes to having a bit of the other in pregnancy, we are all different. Some of us will find those free-flowing pregnancy hormones get us in the mood more often than before. Others will completely lose their mojo and shut up shop the moment they discover they are pregnant. Whatever your feelings are on the matter, it's good to know that unless there are complications (see opposite), sex in pregnancy is totally safe. If you can get to a point where your body and mind can relax, it can also have some really positive benefits for you and your partner. Not only can getting fruity with each other give you time to connect as a couple, it may also help you, mum-to-be, sleep better and increase your happy hormones, thus being a brilliant, natural mood-booster!

Also know that if your partner is male, their penis will **not** prod your baby's head during sex (regardless of what they might think). Your baby has no idea what is going on while safely cocooned and surrounded by amniotic fluid inside of your uterus, and sex will not affect them in the slightest. And having an orgasm is safe and won't start labour off early, although in later pregnancy it may make your Braxton Hicks tightenings (practice contractions) stronger.

Dos

- Take it slowly and talk to your partner about how you are feeling physically and mentally about intimacy during pregnancy. Be sure to communicate what is enjoyable and what is no longer comfortable.

- Use a chemical-free organic lube if you are experiencing any vaginal dryness, or just need a little more help easing into positions.

- Know that oral sex, masturbation, skin-to-skin connection and light touch massage are all safe alternatives if you want to promote oxytocin (love hormone) and endorphins (happy hormones).

- Do a wee after sex to reduce the chance of getting a urinary tract infection (UTI).

Don'ts

- Don't have penetrative sex if your waters have broken, as there is now a throughway to the baby that can increase the chance of infection.

- Don't have sex if you experience vaginal bleeding, as you will need to be checked out at your maternity unit.

- Avoid penetrative sex if you have a low-lying placenta that is either partly or completely covering your cervix.

- Avoid penetrative sex if there have been any concerns that your cervix has begun opening prematurely.

- If you have experience of pre term labour, discuss with your midwife or obstetrician whether it is safe to have sex.

Gentle suggestions

If you are feeling cautious about penetration, you may unintentionally clench your jaw and grit your teeth as your partner enters. A relaxed jaw has a neurological link-up with your pelvic floor (see page 150), so open your mouth and make a 'Ooooo' sound, just as we encourage in labour. It can help release tension and make sex more enjoyable.

Sex at full term (37–42 weeks)

It is often thought that having sex at full term can help start labour; however, there is no hard evidence this is actually the case. What we do know, though, is that hormones released during sex can, in theory, have an impact on the birthing body. First, semen contains naturally occurring prostaglandins that can help soften and ripen the cervix at the tail-end of pregnancy. Secondly, our favourite birthing hormone, oxytocin, is released during mutually gratifying sex. (In fact, a synthetic version of both these hormones is used during a medical induction.) Ultimately, your body and baby will work together to start labour naturally, but keeping calm and relaxed will encourage your wonderful birthing hormones to rise. Whether that involves nooky is up to you!

OXYTOCIN: THE SHY HORMONE

Oxytocin is known to be a shy hormone. It loves low lighting and calm, safe surroundings. Don't underestimate the power of skin-to-skin and soothing touch when it comes to this bonding and comforting hormone. Whether it be a held hand, or a foot or shoulder rub, you and your partner can work together to help your wonderful oxytocin rocket! Oxytocin is our number-one birthing hormone, so keep yourself and your environment as calm as possible to allow this hormone to thrive.

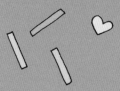

'Lots of my friends always talked about going off sex in pregnancy, but I actually had the opposite response. I'd always been a bit body conscious, and worried about my wobbly bits, so having a beautifully toned round tummy, and bigger boobs than usual, made me feel really amazing. I felt sexy, and loved how I looked.'

EMILY, MUM OF ONE

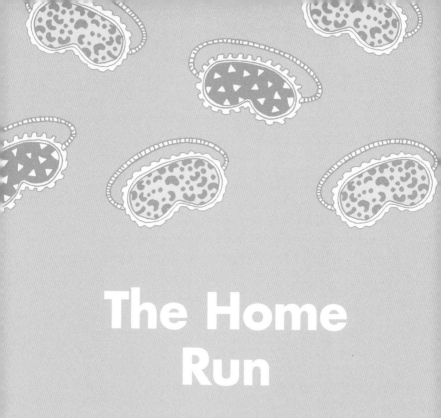

The Home
Run

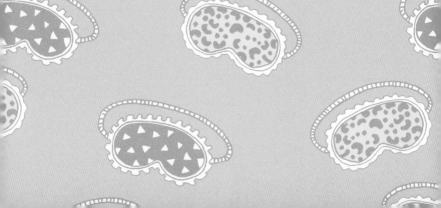

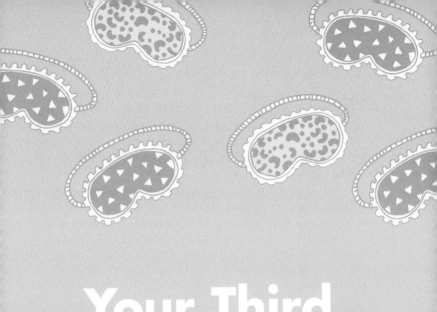

Your Third
Trimester

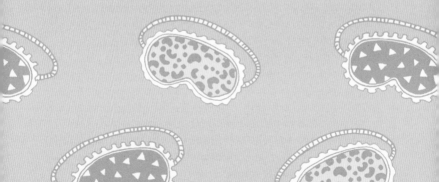

So, here you are heading into the final trimester! This really is an exciting milestone on your journey to motherhood, and a chapter of your pregnancy that can involve feelings of happiness, anticipation and a peppering of nervous energy.

Your bump will be stretching and expanding by the day as your baby is growing stronger and gains more weight, adding to those lovely, cuddly rolls and folds on their little croissant legs.

As your belly continues to grow you may understandably feel more aches, pains and exhaustion, so it is important that you are aware of your limits and listen carefully to your body during this time. In between the shortness of breath as your baby takes up all the space, a strong desire to hire a crane to move you from side to side during the night, and an over-active bladder, you may notice your fatigue and hormones are making you a little more emotional than usual. Talk about how you are feeling with your partner and midwife and be patient and kind with yourself as you head towards your due time.

It's also important to continue and even dial up the self-care during this final trimester to get you in your best shape for birth. You wouldn't try and run a marathon without a bit of training, would you? Luckily, this book has pretty much all the self-care covered for you, so flick back to the nourishing food, gentle stretches, tips and tricks on supporting your body, and practise those calm breathing exercises.

You are getting ever closer to the arrival of your little one, so you may feel ready to start spending some proper time preparing and gathering together the things you and your baby will need in the following months. This is often such an exciting period, when you really start getting your head around the fact that you are about to go through one of life's most incredible experiences.

As always, though, remember you are not a pregnant robot and there is no right or wrong way to approach the final three months of your baby-growing journey. Your third trimester wellbeing is at the core of the following section and we hope these pages help you feel as relaxed and in control as possible as you enter the final weeks of your pregnancy.

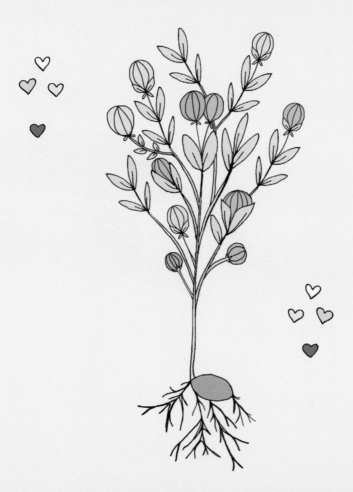

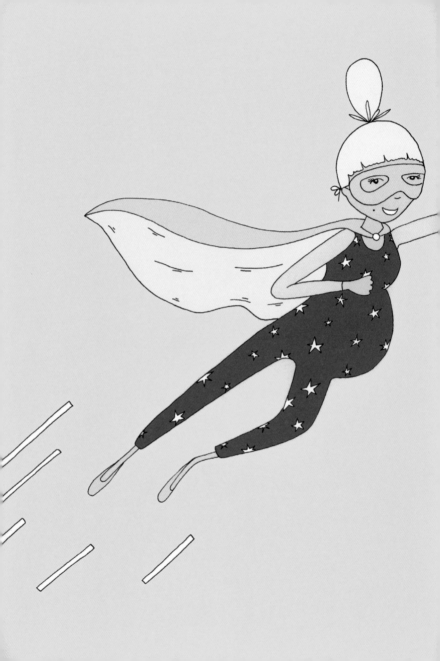

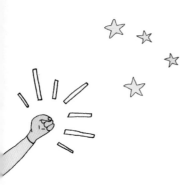

Supporting Your Body Through the Final Trimester

Right now your body is undergoing quite drastic changes, similar to the intensity of the first trimester. Hormones are high, ensuring ligaments are nice and soft to allow baby to move down – and eventually out during birth. As mind-blowing as it is that your body knows how to do this, a not-so-fun side effect is that looser ligaments may mean more aches and pains, and you will really start to feel that extra weight of the bump you are carrying around.

Lots of clients say that they literally feel 'full up' in the third trimester and are concerned that they have no room left for baby to grow. Don't worry: your body has a marvellous capability to keep on expanding even when you think you couldn't possibly give any more!

Being very intentional about how you care for yourself during this time can have a positive impact on how much mental capacity you have to cope with all of these final changes and physical sensations. Remember to treat yourself with love and kindness.

Do at least one of these each day and reap the benefits:

- Go for a walk.

- Have a swim and enjoy the feeling of weightlessness.

- Nourish yourself — eating little and often will probably feel better than three big meals.

- Have a nap or just put your feet up for 5 minutes!

- Get a foot, back or shoulder rub (or see pages 101 and 136 for some self-massage techniques).

- Do 5 minutes of stretching (see pages 138–139).

- Practise your breathwork for 5 minutes (see pages 26 and 130–135).

Little and often has more of an impact on our wellbeing. So 5 minutes each day of doing something caring for yourself will fill up your tank way more than 1 hour each week.

Love lines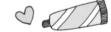

Stretch marks (or, as we like to call them, 'love lines'), may start to appear in the last trimester due to your skin changing shape during the rapid growth of baby and bump. While nothing to worry about, they can sometimes feel a little sore. A gentle massage with coconut oil will help ease discomfort, nourish your skin and relax the muscles, which may help ease any stretching sensations, too. Love lines will usually fade during the postnatal period to a silvery appearance and will be a reminder of the brilliant job you did growing that baby.

The boob lowdown

As you near labour day your breasts will become fuller and heavier, so it'll really help to get yourself a well-fitting bra to support them properly. Try and avoid underwired bras, as the wire can put pressure on your milk ducts. Now's a good time to visit a maternity shop and get measured up for a feeding bra for when your milk comes in, and pack it in your birth bag. You may also find that as your nipples prepare for feeding, they can become a little dry and itchy – moisturise them with a little nut-free oil to keep them soft and itch free.

Where are my ankles?

Swollen feet and ankles can feel sore and achy and leave you in a bit of a pickle with shoe options – we've all been there, unable to wear anything other than flip flops, because our poor feet are so full of fluid. Here are some of our top tips for reducing fluid retention in both your hands and feet:

- Drink more water – we know it feels counterintuitive, but often when we are holding water we actually need to drink more to allow our body to release the excess. Aim for 8–10 small glasses a day.

- Try dandelion leaf tea to help reduce fluid retention.

- Gentle exercise really helps to keep the circulation moving, which will also reduce fluid retention.

- Eat more foods that contain magnesium and potassium – see our Nourishing Grub: Part I section on pages 28–29.

- Have Epsom salt baths to ease the stretched skin and to draw out the excess fluid from the tissues. See page 67.

- Get someone to gently massage your hands and feet in an upward motion toward the heart. This will stimulate the lymphatic system to get to work and remove the excess fluid. The lymph sits under the skin, on top of the muscle, so keep the pressure light.

Potent pineapple

The pineapple is well known as a great source of nutrients, but did you know that the bit we discard has lots of medicinal properties? Pineapple skin contains high concentrates of an enzyme called bromelain, which is used to treat swelling and inflammation of the body. Reported to have been used in South and Central America since the 1800s, it is also a great digestive aid, and is said to help ease symptoms of constipation, IBS and upset tummies.

HOW TO MAKE SOOTHING PINEAPPLE SKIN TEA

1. Give the pineapple a wash, then slice off the skin — keep the flesh to eat later on.

2. Place all the skin in a large saucepan with 2 cinnamon sticks and a chunk of fresh root ginger. Cover with 1 litre of boiling water and allow to simmer for 30 minutes, topping up the water if needed. Take off the heat and allow to steep for another 30 minutes.

3. Drain the tea through a sieve and serve hot or cold. You can keep this tea in the fridge for up to 3 days. Drink 1–2 cups a day until symptoms reduce.

Backache

As your back muscles work hard to support your growing bump, you may find yourself experiencing backache more often. Get your partner or a friend to look at the back massage section on pages 102–103, and use some soothing essential oils to give you a lovely aches-and-pains-busting rub down.

Instructions for your partner/friend:

1. We suggest adding 1 drop of black pepper essential oil and 2 drops of bergamot or sweet orange essential oil to 15ml of grapeseed oil. Mix together well.

2. Using your essential oil blend, follow the back massage instructions on pages 102–103 to relax the back muscles and ease backache for your lovely mum-to-be.

3. Cat-cow (see page 64) is a lovely stretch to engage those tummy muscles and really ease and relieve an overworked, achy back.

Bounce

Now is a good time to up the use of the birthing ball. Sitting on a birthing ball rather than a sofa is a great way to engage your abdominal muscles, giving them a workout and keeping them strong. It also encourages you to sit in the perfect posture for optimal baby positioning, which will help with birthing baby more easily.

A Pain in the Bum

A common but uncomfortable side effect of the third trimester can be haemorrhoids, or piles. These are swollen veins around or inside the lower rectum. They can feel sore and itchy, and if very inflamed can bleed a little after a bowel movement. But don't worry, they are easy to treat and will usually go away on their own a little while after birth.

Cooling pads

Like any inflammation, piles can be soothed by a cold compress, which can take away the heat and itchiness and often help reduce them in size. You can make your own soothing cold compresses at home very easily.

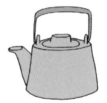

1. Place 4 chamomile tea bags in a big heatproof jug, cover with boiling water and leave to steep for 30 minutes.

2. Grab some of your big maternity pads (if you don't have them yet, use normal sanitary pads, or even a few clean washcloths). Place them on a baking tray. If using pads, place them waterproof-side down in the tray; washcloths should be loosely rolled into a sausage shape.

3. You can use tea alone, or for extra help add a glug of
    witch hazel and a cup of Epsom salts to the jug of tea.
    If you'd like to use some essential oils, add 2 drops each
    of lavender (soothing) and tea tree (antibacterial) to the
    Epsom salts before you add them. Mix well, pour over the
    pads or washcloths until they are saturated, then place the
    tray in the fridge to cool the pads for a couple of hours.

4. To use, place a thick towel or waterproof sheet down on
    your chair or sofa, place a pad or washcloth against the
    sore area (you might have to push it into place so that it's
    between the cheeks and against the anus) and enjoy the
    cooling relief for at least 15 minutes. Dispose of the pad
    or add the washcloth to the washing pile. Dry yourself
    gently with a clean towel and if you have any protruding
    piles, now's a good time to pop them back in (see below).

Push them back in

If your piles are protruding outside of your bottom, the
sensitive tissue that is used to being on the inside of your body
will now be rubbing against your underwear and skin, causing
irritation and inflammation. The best thing to do is to gently
pop them back inside the anus. Do this after using the cooling
pads (above) or after each bowel movement (after cleansing
with a wipe or quick sitz bath).

With freshly washed fingers, add a little oil (you can just
use olive oil from the kitchen) to your anus. Then gently guide
the pile back inside. Don't over-push it, and leave it if it really
hurts, but usually it'll pop back in easily. You should feel much
better with it back inside and the swelling should subside
more quickly, free from irritation. If they are causing a lot of
discomfort, talk to your GP about using a medicated cream.

Staying Regular!

There are many reasons we may become a bit bunged up in pregnancy, causing gas and bloating and leaving you feeling a bit uncomfortable. Here are our top tips for staying regular:

- **Stay hydrated.** Steering clear of caffeinated drinks (these actually act as diuretics and dehydrate the body) really helps, as does drinking your fluids from a bottle or large glass so that you can mentally take note of how much is going in. The colon needs water to do its job, so lack of it can be a big cause of constipation.

- **Eat wiser.** Foods that can help keep you regular are: prunes, apples, pears, kiwi fruit, figs, green leafy veg, rhubarb, sweet potato, beans, peas, lentils, chia seeds and flaxseeds.

PLEASE NOTE: Remember that every time you increase the fibre in your diet you will need to increase your fluid intake, too. This enables the fibre to absorb the fluid and pass through the digestive tract smoothly.

- **Increase magnesium intake.** Magnesium is not only great for the muscles and the nervous system, it's also great for our gut health. You can naturally increase your magnesium intake by adding Epsom salts to your bath, or by using a magnesium spray on the soles of your feet at bedtime. If you want to take a magnesium supplement make sure you do so under the guidance of a nutritionist so that you know you are taking the right amount for your body. Or, eat more magnesium-rich foods (see page 30).

- **Start the day with hot water and lemon.** A mug of hot water with a slice of lemon is a great way to start the day. The citric acid in the lemon acts as a gentle, natural laxative, fighting toxins in the digestive tract and flushing them out of your body more easily. High in vitamin C, it can also help with indigestion.

- **Breathe.** Sometimes we are backed up because we are frazzled and this has put our body into 'fight or flight' mode. When our stressors are stimulated our muscles constrict and this doesn't allow for an easy 'release'. Breathing is a great tool to help the body to 'let go' and to encourage our stress hormones to lower.

- **While sitting on the toilet,** take some big, slow breaths in and out and allow all of the muscles in your body to relax and let go. After a few minutes you should feel the anus muscles relaxing enough to allow release. This will help you not to strain, which can cause or aggravate uncomfortable haemorrhoids in pregnancy.

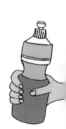

- **Try liquid iron.** If you do need to take iron supplements (which can cause constipation), you could speak to your healthcare provider about trying liquid iron such as Spatone, which is less cloggy than iron in tablet form, and may be worth trying first.

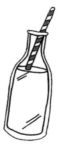
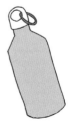

Third Trimester Headspace

It is understandable that up until the final few months of your pregnancy you have been busy living your day-to-day life and perhaps have regarded the arrival of your baby as something ahead of you and too abstract to really spend any length of time contemplating in detail.

Now, you find yourself on the last leg of your pregnancy journey and the undeniable presence of your little lodger kicking away in there, teamed up with other people's curiosities surrounding when your bump will turn into a baby, makes you realise they will be here before you know it and you may not be sure if you are mentally ready for such a significant life change!

Holding some time back for yourself to really think about where you are at in your headspace and how you hope to prepare for this brand new human and the changes their arrival will make in your life can benefit you hugely, and help you feel calmer, more focused and organised as you navigate your way through your final trimester.

1. **Give your mind air-time.** It is very common to experience waves of anxiety and feel overwhelmed during this period as your brain tries to pre-empt what is about to happen to your body and your life. Your thoughts may become preoccupied by birth and your baby's wellbeing. Do communicate your worries and talk them through with your partner, friends and even your midwife. Their reassurance and understanding can be enough to help lighten the mental load that you are carrying around with you and will remind you that you are not alone during this significant life transition.

2. **Time for bed.** Once again we come back to rest, but that's because it really is so important, and exhaustion has a lot to answer for when it comes to exacerbating anything that may be troubling you. A tiny tadpole of a worry can grow into a big frightening warty toad in the dark, quiet hours of a sleepless night. An overactive mind can even filter through into your dreams as you subconsciously play out your worries around giving birth and concerns for your baby. Turn to our guidance and ideas for how to get the best night's sleep and try to have some downtime before bed (see pages 80–83), practise your breathwork and/or use the partner relaxation script on pages 126–129 to help you wind down before you hit the hay.

3. **Identity shake-up.** When a baby is born, a mother is born also. It is very normal that you will spend some time during the final months thinking about who you will become once your baby arrives. Sometimes this may leave you feeling confused and even a little lost as to what this identity shift will mean for you. The bottom line is that you will still be you, with the extra layer of motherhood around you. Don't expect too much of yourself and trust the process, because when your baby arrives you will find a new groove that works for you and your family set-up, and part of that comes from approaching your new role with curiosity and flexibility.

4. **The other half.** If you have a partner you may have both found yourselves wondering how your baby is going to change your family dynamic. Life is busy and if you have been going to bed early you may have felt like ships that pass in the night, with both of you having a lot on your mind. A new baby is a life-changing event and it's

important to get away from your daily routine to spend some quality undisturbed time connecting with each other emotionally and mentally. Some couples plan an actual babymoon, where they either spend some intentional time together at home or away talking, planning, resting and nurturing a little romance in preparation for their baby's arrival. Even if you don't do that, make time to talk to each other about how you are both feeling, and connect with each other as a couple.

5. **Go slow.** It is very natural to start to focus inwards during your pregnancy, especially during the final months. Once again, return to your instinct. If life feels too hectic and fast and you are longing to spend more time quietly preparing your mind and nesting at home in your own company, then try to respond to that internal request where possible. By doing this when you can, you'll be able to calm your busy thoughts, which in turn can leave you feeling more mentally prepared as you approach your due time (37–42 weeks).

The relaxation (oxytocin- and endorphin-releasing) script

This little script, opposite, is perfect for your birthing partner to read to you during pregnancy and labour. It is a simple but effective way of connecting with one another and promoting a calm state of mind, encouraging those powerful birthing hormones to thrive and respond to any bubbling adrenaline that might be present. Light touch is so effective at stimulating both oxytocin and endorphins, so let's get cosy, dim the lights and get started.

Birth partner to sit opposite mum-to-be. Mum-to-be place your hand in your partner's lap, palm facing the ceiling. Sleeve rolled up to the elbow.

Partner to read the following (calmly, quietly and slowly):

1

Take a few moments to close your eyes, relax your jaw and shoulders and take three slow, refreshing breaths, in through your nose and out through your mouth... (pause for three breaths).

2

It's time to let go of any tension from your body and enjoy feeling calm and at peace. Just focus on my words and know that we are here together in this moment and I am by your side.

3

Take your attention to the top of your head and consciously release any tension from your scalp, and deeply relax (pause for 5 seconds).

4

Now focus on your forehead and release any tension that may be present, and deeply relax (pause).

5

Move your attention to your eyebrows and eyes and let them fully relax, releasing any tightness from the little muscles around your brows and eyes (pause).

6 Feel how good it is to let all that tension slip away, comfortable and deeply relaxed (pause).

7 Move your attention to your jaw and let relaxation unlock any clenched or gritted teeth as it washes over you, leaving you deeply relaxed (pause).

8 Now move to the back of your head and neck and release any tension, deeply relaxed (pause).

9 Gently soften and release tension that may be held in your neck and tops of your shoulders, deeply relax (pause). (Now start slowly circling your fingers around the palm of your partner's hand.)

10 When you let go of the tightness and tension, you can feel the oxygen flowing freely and easily through your body, carrying those important birthing hormones to where they need to be.

11 As you feel my soft touch, imagine your oxytocin flowing throughout your body and into your uterus, encouraging the squeezing and releasing like a mesh wrapping itself around the muscle fibres, as your body does exactly what it needs to do to bring you (us) closer to meeting your (our) baby.

12 Know that you are doing so well as you release tension, let go and breathe through these powerful physical sensations.

13 (Now start moving your fingers up the forearm and to the arm crease, then return down to the wrist, continue back and forth.)

14 Let your concentration follow my fingers as they trace up and down your arm. No need to focus on any other physical sensation, just my touch and these words.

15 Notice how your birthing body knows what to do as you let go and breathe through each wave of sensation. Calm, relaxed and in control (pause).

16 Now focus on the endorphins that are working for your benefit, rising and growing in strength to help keep you comfortable; your body's clever way to ease and relieve strong and powerful sensations, perfectly designed to ease and relieve your body as you (we) get closer to meeting your (our) baby.

17 Now, bring your attention back to your breath, and take three more deep breaths in through your nose and out through your mouth (pause).

PLEASE NOTE: If mum-to-be wishes to remain deeply relaxed and would rather you continue, then just loop round to the beginning again.

18 Know that you are strong and in control during every contraction and that those powerful sensations have purpose and are carrying you towards your baby. As we come full circle know that I will remain by your side throughout and we can intentionally focus on releasing tension and encouraging a surge of birthing hormones whenever you need.

19 Continue to release and relax your shoulders, move your attention outside of your body, stretch and open your eyes slowly…

Breathwork for Birth

The more you carve out the time to practise your breathwork for birth, the more quickly you will be able to calm any fast, shallow adrenaline-fuelled breathing that may occur from time to time during pregnancy and labour. Although your day-to-day breathing is an unconscious physical activity, it really is possible and powerful to control and regulate your own inhale/exhale cycle. By using some very simple techniques you can effectively calm down that unhelpful bubbling adrenaline. This in turn will have a wonderful effect on your oxytocin and endorphin levels, helping you let go of any unwelcome tension and tightness in your birthing body so you feel more relaxed and in control. A good flow of oxygen is also very important to help your baby remain content as they go through the strong squeezing and releasing of labour with you, and our uterus needs a good oxygen supply to work as efficiently as possible.

Are you dancing or fighting with your body?

We always get our mums-to-be to do this little activity, just to reinforce how important it is to let go of physical tension and breathe consciously through episodes of strong and powerful sensations.

(A) Set your phone timer for 60 seconds and stand upright, feet hip-width apart. Gently drop your bottom into a squat (be careful not to go too deep or you may lose your balance). Now start your timer and clench. Really grit your teeth, jaw, neck and shoulders and buttocks. Don't think about your breathing (although you may find you feel like holding your

breath or breathing quickly with all that tension in your body).
When 60 seconds are up, release and relax.

Take a minute's break

(B) Now set your 60-second timer again. Stand upright, feet
hip-width apart. Gently drop into a squat again. This time we
want you to be very intentional with your breathing. Close
your eyes, consciously relax your teeth, jaw, neck, shoulders
and buttocks. Breathe in through your nose, in a relaxed
and controlled way, then make an 'O' with your lips, blowing
the air slowly away while making a calm audible 'Ooooo'
sound. Sway your hips from side to side as your legs and bum
feel heavier. Continue until the 60 seconds are up.

You are likely to have noticed that during (A) you felt a lot
less comfortable and more aware of the length of time. Your
tension and your lack of control regarding your breathing
meant you were 'fighting' against your body while feeling
discomfort. During (B) you may have felt more in control,
allowing your body to move and 'dance' to counterbalance
those strong sensations. This can leave us feeling more
relaxed, which can help gently move that physical tension,
and by being more focused on our breathing technique, we
are encouraging oxygen to be delivered to our muscles and
will often feel less discomfort during that squat.

So how can we learn to dance with the strong sensations
we will experience during labour? The trick is keeping your
breathing techniques as SIMPLE as possible during labour and
birth. There really is no need for bells and whistles: easy and
effective is what we are looking for here to ensure you gently
guide your breathing in the right direction.

1. Diaphragmatic breathing

Deep breathing can help you to expend less energy (saving it for when you need it the most), lower your heart rate and blood pressure and help you tolerate the strong physical sensations of birthing more effectively. It is the opposite of shallow adrenaline-fuelled chest breathing.

For evidence that you are getting that breath to where it needs to be, place your hand flat, palm against your tummy, above your belly button. With your in-breath you should notice your abdomen expand and push your hand gently outwards. When you breathe out, your hand will descend back again to its starting position. Think of your belly as a balloon that you are carefully blowing up on the in-breath, then releasing the air from slowly on the out-breath.

In established labour (4–10cm), the strong squeezing, releasing and pushing sensations of contractions are likely to be present around a third of the time, coming and going rhythmically in waves. Use your breathwork to ease you through your contractions, and don't forget to rest between each one.

2. The 'opening' breath

It makes sense to use a breathing technique that complements what you are feeling during a contraction. The 'opening' breathing technique works in harmony with your uterus during labour, as your cervix moves forward, thins out and opens right up until the point of full dilatation (10cm dilated). Practise this opening breath twice a day throughout the third trimester, or any time you feel anxious and in need of some calm. If this breath took roughly 12 seconds per cycle, then you could aim for around 5 breaths to carry you through your contraction.

- Sit or stand comfortably.

- Relax your shoulders and close your eyes.

- Be mindful to release tension in your jaw and shoulders.

- Breathe in through your nose for 4 slow counts.

- Breathe out through your mouth for 8 slow counts.

- If counting your breaths makes you feel uncomfortable or dizzy, then just trace your mind's eye around a rectangle shape (a door is a good image to visualise) so that the in-breath travels along the short side and the out-breath travels along the long side.

- Visualise your cervix gently and carefully opening up with each strong sensation.

- If you would rather a visualisation not linked to your birthing body, imagine on the out-breath blowing a big bubble that slowly moves up into the air, or releasing the string of a kite until it is flying high above you (or any image that complements the pulling up and opening of your cervix).

3. The releasing breath

Once your cervix has reached full dilatation then the sensation of birthing changes and so can your breathing in order to support the 'bearing down' feeling that is often compared to the sensation of needing to go for a poo. The cervix is now fully dilated and is no longer holding the baby back and in position. The muscular fibres of the uterus change their tact and push your little one down into the vagina to release your baby for birth.

- Sit or stand comfortably.

- Relax shoulders and close your eyes.

- Be mindful to release tension in your jaw and shoulders.

- Breathe in through your nose slowly to the count of 5. Breathe slowly and audibly, as though you are exaggerating the sniffing of flowers.

- Breathe out slowly and controlled through your nose, again to the count of 5.

- If counting your breaths makes you feel uncomfortable or dizzy, then slowly trace your mind's eye around a square shape, even on each side.

- Visualise the top of your uterus pushing your baby down with each strong sensation.

- Or imagine with your out-breath a powerful waterfall flowing downwards, leaves falling from a tree, snow floating to the ground or any other visualisation that complements your baby moving down through the open cervix and being released.

- Make that out-breath audible and imagine the air travelling down from your nose and through your body like a wave, releasing your baby into the birth canal (when in labour try not to hold your breath unless otherwise instructed by your midwife or doctor).

- Trust that your uterus knows what it is doing, let go physically and breathe your baby down.

Midwives will often talk about the sensation of birthing being comparable to doing the biggest poo of your life, and that is because both birth and doing a poo require your body to bear down, with a squeezing down and releasing motion. For this reason, it may be useful to practise your 'releasing breath' technique on the loo every time you do a poo. Don't strain, just gently breathe and let go.

And on that note…as baby pushes down, the pressure on the rectum can cause you to pass a little poo – this is completely normal and in fact we get very excited by it as it means baby is making its way down. Do not worry, your midwife will be very subtle at getting rid of it before you even know about it!

massages + stretches

As your gorgeous baby continues to grow, and your body expands to accommodate it, you will require a little more TLC to help ease the aches and pains these changes may bring.

> PLEASE NOTE: never massage over the bone, only on the muscles — and in pregnancy avoid massaging too deeply into the middle of the tops of the shoulders and the inside of the ankles, where there are some acupressure points that can stimulate labour.

JAW MASSAGE

There is a weird and wonderful neurological link-up between the jaw and vagina muscles, so it's important to start getting that tension out of your jaw in the third trimester; this will also help with neck tension and headaches, and stop you clenching your teeth at night. Every morning and evening when you apply your moisturiser, massage into the big muscle at the sides of your jaw. Clench your teeth, and find the muscle that bulges out at the sides of your jaw (the masseter muscle). Place your fingers on each side, release your teeth and massage into the muscle in little circular motions.

TENNIS BALL RUB-DOWN

The feedback we often have is that partners can often be a little rough, and massage a bit too deeply with their thumbs. If this is the case for you then worry not, we've got just the answer. Grab a trusty tennis ball (preferably a clean, new one) get comfy, and ask your partner, friend or family member to roll the ball in little circles over your tight spots. Using a tennis ball is a great way to keep the pressure firm enough, but not painful. Guide them to the areas where you are feeling tight (also see page 101).

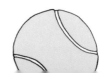

SINUS MASSAGE

Hormone changes can result in you feeling more bunged up and stuffy (almost like having a cold or hay fever) and can also be a trigger for those horrid hormonal headaches around your eyes and forehead. This self-massage technique is a fab way to release tension, encourage sinus drainage, clear your stuffy nose and ease headache symptoms. This may cause the nose to run a little, so have a tissue to hand.

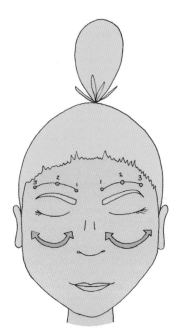

1. Using your thumb or middle finger (thumb for more pressure, middle finger for less) press into points 1, 2 and 3. Press in, hold for the count of 5, release, then move along to the next point. Repeat a few times.

2. Using your middle fingers, press into either side of the bridge of your nose and, keeping the pressure constant, trace under the cheekbones and out towards your ears, following the line of the sinuses. Repeat a few times.

A GOOD-OLD FOOT RUB

Nothing beats a good old-fashioned foot rub, especially in the third trimester when arches can collapse a little as your muscles relax and your bump gets heavier, and there may be a little water retention in the ankles too. We have found from experience that if your partner watches TV while they massage, they are distracted and massage for longer! Definitely worth a try! Next time you settle down to watch TV, casually pop a foot up on their lap - hopefully that'll be all the hint they need!

HIP-RELIEVING STRETCH

All that side sleeping and extra mobility in the pelvis can cause a bit of tightness and stiffening up in the hips and glutes. This wonderful hip stretch doesn't put any pressure on the groin and is safe for anyone with pubis pain to do.

Do this stretch while the kettle is boiling; that way you are likely to do it at least a couple of times a day without even thinking!

1. Stand upright beside the kitchen table or counter, but stand a little away from it, with both feet together.

2. Lean your upper body towards the table, and push your hips away from it - hold for the count of 10. Keep your outside leg straight and your inside leg slightly bent.

3. Repeat on the other side.

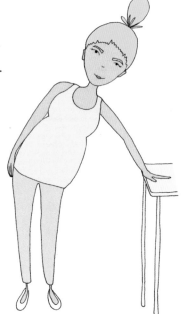

GAS–RELIEVING STRETCH

Ladies, it's totally normal to be a little gassier than usual in pregnancy, but it can be a little uncomfortable. This is a fab stretch to lengthen the digestive tract and compress the bowels a little to help air to pass a little more easily. This can result in gas being passed from either end, so you may want to do this one in private - unless you are happy expelling gas in company, in which case good on you!

1. Place a pillow on the floor and then position yourself on your hands and knees, with your head near the pillow.

2. Move your knees as close to your chest as your bump allows and then lower your head down on to the pillow, keeping your bottom up in the air. Breathe normally.

3. Stay like this for a minute, then turn your head to the other side and rest for a further minute (longer if you like - just keep turning the head so that you don't get a crook neck).

4. Repeat whenever you feel the need!

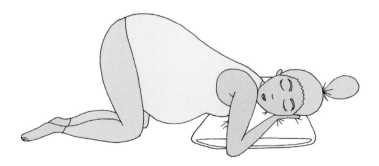

yoga for the
third trimester

Yoga is a great way to prepare the mind and body for labour. We've seen lots of our ladies ease many a third trimester ailment with regular pregnancy yoga practice. We have also noticed that women who have practised breathwork and meditation regularly during pregnancy are better able to keep calm during labour. Here, one of our favourite yoga teachers, Kiranjot, shares her favourite birth-prep yoga tools.

9-minute meditation to relieve stress

As wonderful as being pregnant is, it can also bring with it stress and anxiety. This practice relieves the pressure of stress by clearing the space of the heart so you can think and feel more clearly. You can do this cross-legged on the floor or in a chair; just make sure you are sitting straight and your feet are flat on the floor.

This meditation is done in three parts, allowing 3 minutes for each section.

Step 1: For 3 minutes

- Press the thumb and index finger of your left hand together and rest your hand on your knee.

- Bend your right arm at the elbow with the forearm crossing the body, palm facing down.

- Like a windscreen wiper, you are going to move the forearm up and down powerfully from the belly button to the third eye (that magical space between your eyebrows of intuition) with long, deep breaths.

- Close your eyes and focus your mind's eye on the very centre of your chin, which helps keep your emotions in check.

- After 1 minute make a fist with your left hand with your thumb inside and squeeze it hard, this will keep your ego in check.

- Stop at 3 minutes and take a couple of deep breaths as you relax your arms back down to your knees.

Step 2: For 3 minutes

- Keeping elbows bent, bring both arms out to the front, left palm down, right palm facing up, and close your eyes.

- Bounce your forearms up and down – like the big juggling act of life. Eyes stay closed and focused at the centre of the chin.

- Stop at 3 minutes and take a couple of deep breaths as you relax your arms back down to your knees.

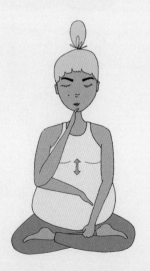
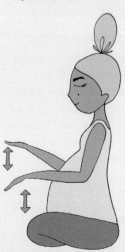

Step 3: For 3 minutes

- Close your eyes and place your hands right over left over your heart chakra (the centre of your chest). Tilt your head left and right slowly.

- Inhale left, exhale right.

- Keep your eyes closed and focused at the very centre of your chin.

- After 2 minutes take a deep breath in, straighten your neck and stretch your arms up as high as you can.

- Hold with long, deep breathing for 1 minute then relax your arms down and leave your hands upturned in your lap. Relax your body and rest for as many breaths as you need.

- Use a timer to learn what a minute feels like when you are using active breath control. This is a

great practice for labour, as surges typically last a minute. If you learn to calm your breath for 60 seconds this will really help you during birth.

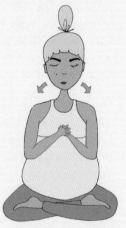

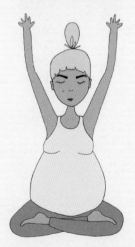

Meditation to conquer pain

This next practice is a challenge that will help you develop your tolerance to interesting sensations like labour surges. Start at 3 minutes and try building up to 11! Give yourself a powerful experience of strength you never knew you had.

- Make Spock hands (the thumb extended and the fingers touching, but parted between the middle finger and ring finger) and extend your arms out to the sides. Really stretch them, long and strong. Left palm faces down, right palm faces up.

- Keep softening your face and shoulders throughout the meditation.

- With your eyes open, focus your gaze to the tip of your nose, keep it there for the whole length of the meditation.

- Suck the breath in deep through your mouth and exhale powerfully through your nose. See if you can control your breath the whole way through.

- Aim for 8 breaths a minute, which is roughly in for a count of 4 and out for 4. You can count it out in your head or silently use a mantra. We use Sat Nam in Kundalini, it's a mantra for your soul.

Sat Nam means truth is my identity. Breathe in Sat, exhale Nam.

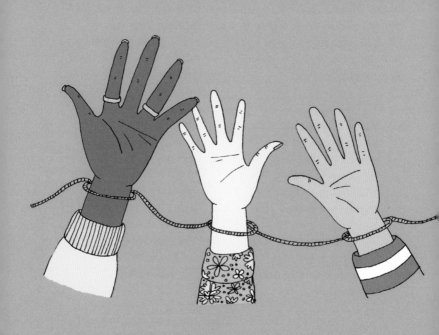

Cultural Rituals and Traditions for Mum-to-be

In our current Western set-up people are often living away from family, with very busy lives. During times of big change, a lack of community and connection can feel very isolating. More and more women are nowadays turning back to rituals, traditions and ceremonies around pregnancy, birth and the postnatal period in an attempt to feel more supported and connected to other women around them.

A gathering of community and celebration of mum-to-be is a tradition that is still very present in many cultures, and as a result women often face birth feeling more supported and cared for. Living in extended communities means a sharing of stories and knowledge and this can be comforting for a new mother as she approaches birth.

- In Zimbabwe, expectant mothers go home and stay with their family a few weeks before their birth. Here they rest and are fed special nourishing foods and drinks to prepare them for labour.

- In India, mothers have a type of baby shower after the seventh month called a 'Godh Bharai' – this ceremony celebrates the mum-to-be and showers her with blessings, gifts, nourishing foods and prayers.

- In Polynesia, an expectant mum is treated like a goddess and is pampered by her entire community. She is waited on while she rests and her midwife visits often and gives her regular massages!

- A tradition that is being used more and more in Western culture is a version of the Navajo Blessingway – a ceremony that celebrates a mother before her child is born. It can be a wonderful way to catch up with all of your friends before birth and to fill yourself up with all their love and support. In the UK, this celebration of the mother is mainly organised in one of two ways:

1. **A Baby Shower,** which is organised a little like a hen party. This is usually a party, or sometimes a lunch or dinner with party games and gifts, and is a chance for the mum-to-be to get together with all of her friends and family before she has her baby. It provides a chance for friends and family to wish her well and shower her with gifts, which are often for the baby.

2. **A Mother Blessing** is more a celebration of mum-to-be, and a celebration of her approaching birth. It is a get-together with all the expectant mum's special female friends and family, and the focus is very much on her and not the baby. All the guests bring food for the day, birth offerings and gifts for the mother and she is pampered and nourished, with the focus being on building a supportive community for birth and beyond.

Ceremonies and Rituals

Red thread

The red thread is a beautiful ritual, that literally ties mum-to-be to her community! At your celebration, gather all of the women together in a circle. One person takes the lead, and with a ball of red thread (and a pair of scissors in their pocket, otherwise you may become stuck!) she starts with mum-to-be and wraps the thread three times around her wrist, then she moves on to the other women, wrapping the thread three times around one wrist of each woman in turn, until she comes back to the expectant mum. As the women all sit connected, they each say a wish for their friend, offer up a piece of advice, or share a supportive story. The thread is then cut and each woman's thread is tied into a bracelet (make sure you secure it well – it may be on for a while). This bracelet is then worn by all the women, until they receive news of baby's safe arrival.

During labour, every time mum-to-be looks down at her wrist, she will feel the love and support of all those who were joined to her during her ceremony.

Birth necklace

Similar to the red thread ritual above, some people choose to have a birth necklace made at their mother celebration. They ask each woman who attends to find one bead that makes them think of the expectant mum, they each then bring this bead with them to the Mother Blessing or Baby Shower. The host supplies a necklace cord that is long enough to fit over mum-to-be's head, and then one by one, each guest takes it in turn to share the bead, explain why it made them think of their friend, and then string it on to the cord. The necklace is then tied and placed over mum-to-be's head, ready for her to wear on her labour day. The idea is that it is a tactile and visual reminder of her support network, all rooting for her during birth.

Birth letters

A wonderful birth ritual we have seen a few times now, and that brings us to tears every time, are birth letters. These are letters written to you by your most special people – ask them

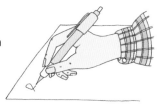

to write you words of love and encouragement, that might give you a lovely lift that you can read during labour should you need a little boosting pep talk! We think these are a beautiful way of giving a birthing mama a huge hit of oxytocin when she'll need it the most. Once you have them, keep them sealed (no peeking) and pop them in your birth bag ready for the big day. Tell your birth partner where they are so that they can grab them for you when they feel you might need them during labour.

Day 3 jar

Day 3 can be a tricky day for a new mum. It's around this day the oxytocin high crashes down and the hormones that bring the milk in soar, often bringing with them lots of tears. These hormones can make us feel very low and it is not uncommon for mums to feel very weepy on this day. The Day 3 jar is a little jar full of little words of love and encouragement from friends and family, all written on paper, folded up and popped in the jar for mum to read when she needs a little lift on Day 3. This is a good one for a friend to organise for you – get them to ask friends and family to email messages over to her, and then she can make up the jar for you and give it to you at your mother celebration.

Labour candle

This is another ritual that connects women together to support the birthing mum. Buy a job-lot of lovely candles, then give them as a little gift to each of the women who attend your Baby Shower, or Mother Blessing, keeping one back for yourself. The idea behind the labour candle is that you will light your candle when labour begins and then send out a message to all of your 'candle gang' who will then light their candle, too.

A client of ours who did this said that it was so comforting while she was in labour to think of lots of little flickers of light spread around town, all in honour of her and her birth day. Remember, though, that you don't want lots of people messaging you while you are labouring, so make sure that your ladies know to light their candle and then leave you to it.

Jaws, Straws and Vaginas!

One of our favourite wacky facts is the bizarre neurological link-up between the jaw and the sphincter muscles – namely the vagina and anus muscles. If you are tightly clenched in your jaw, chances are you'll be tightly clenched down there, too – and this is not going to help you during labour when these muscles need to soften and stretch to allow your baby to make its way down and out into the world.

You may think that you don't clench your jaw, but you'll be surprised how many of us do it without even realising. But don't worry! There are some very quick and easy ways to ensure that you keep the clenching in check. And this is where the straws come into play.

First, they are just plain old practical. You'll need lots of sips of water throughout labour to keep hydrated. As labour progresses you may find yourself in funny positions which can sometimes make drinking a little tricky. Pop a reusable bendy straw in the glass or bottle and, hey presto, you can drink in whatever position you need to.

The second wonder of the straw is its action of loosening the jaw. When you suck through a straw, the shape you have to make with your mouth actually releases the jaw. Every time you take a sip of fluid you will naturally release the tension in your jaw without even thinking about it.

Another lovely way to keep that jaw nice and relaxed is to get into the habit of massaging the masseter muscle (see page 136). Finally, opening your mouth: yawning, wiggling your jaw from side to side and blowing raspberries can all help. So, there you have it! A little prep work with the jaw can help you tremendously in the run up to and through labour. If in doubt, think FLOPPY FACE = FLOPPY FANNY.

Preparing for Birth

Birth plans

We agree: it really is quite impossible to plan birth, and getting too hung up on a rigid plan of how you would like birth to go can actually cause more harm mentally and emotionally for a mum-to-be than good. However, making a rough plan for something enables us to put time into thinking about it. It allows us to explore our options and feel a bit more in control. We tend to tackle the birth-plan problem by encouraging couples to write a Plan A, B and C. This way they can feel calm and prepared for whatever might happen.

PLAN A is your wish list. If everything went smoothly, what would this birth look like for you?

PLAN B is what happens if you need to transfer into hospital from a home birth, or from the midwife-led unit to labour ward. Or, perhaps you are already on the labour ward and need some extra assistance. Understanding what this change of plan and environment will roughly look like can settle worries and anxieties, and afford a sense of calm should Plan B need to be engaged.

PLAN C is your in-case-of-an-emergency C-section birth plan. We know that birth is unpredictable, but rest assured you will have a fabulous team of healthcare professionals monitoring you and baby to keep you safe.

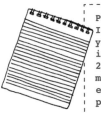

PREPARING FOR AN ELECTIVE C-SECTION
If you are planning an elective C-section you will find lots of self-care advice in our abdominal birth section on pages 209–211. We suggest you take a look and make a list of all the ways that you can enhance your comfort and care as you prepare for the birth of your baby.

Some questions to ask yourself to help write your birth plan:

- Who do you want with you in the birth room?

- Where would you like to give birth? On the bed, in water, standing…

- Will your partner cut the cord, announce the sex, hand you the baby?

- Would you like delayed cord clamping and immediate skin-to-skin?

- Would you like music? Who will make a playlist?

- Would you like photos taken? These can be for your eyes only, and can be very lovely to look back on.

- Do you have religious needs that you'd like your birth team to work with?

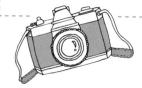

Remember that oxytocin! Anything that makes you feel calm and safe will be good for you in labour. Add it all on to the birth plan – low lighting, warmth, soft music, whatever makes you feel great!

In your birth plan, also note down things you wouldn't like or if there is anything you find triggering. Perhaps you have a needle phobia, or you find internal examinations upsetting, or perhaps you've had a bad experience in a hospital and you are a little anxious about going in again. All of this information is really helpful for your birth team, so they know how best to look after you so that you feel truly supported.

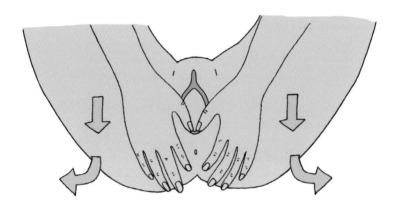

Preparing the perineum

Perineal massage helps to soften the tissues of the perineum
and get them used to the stretching sensation of birth.
Performing the massage daily from 35 weeks can help to
lengthen the muscle fibres, allowing a better stretch.

You can do the massage in the bath where the warm
water will also help to soften the tissue, or after a bath or
shower, reclined on your bed using some natural oil such as
coconut or grapeseed. Make sure you are nice and relaxed
before you start the massage; tense muscles are more
sensitive, so try taking some nice deep breaths before you
begin. And make sure that your hands and fingernails are
clean before you massage.

Don't try perineal massage if you think you may have a
vaginal infection or if your waters may have broken. If
anything feels too uncomfortable don't continue, and seek
further advice from your midwife.

1. Sit or lean back in a comfortable position.

2. Put your thumbs just inside the vagina (no more than 2.5cm, or up to your first knuckle nearest your nail).

3. Press down towards your anus and then to the sides until you feel a slight burning, stinging, or tingling sensation.

4. Hold this stretch for 1–2 minutes.

5. Now, gently massage the lower bit of your vagina. Using your thumbs, slide them outwards and upwards and then back again in a U-shaped movement. Continue this for no longer than 2–3 minutes. You could practise your slow, deep breathing techniques while you do this (see page 132).

6. You may get to a point where it becomes hard to reach your own perineum and you may need to enlist the help of your birth partner.

7. Simply follow the same method as before. The only difference is that your partner should use their index fingers rather than thumbs to perform side-to-side and U-shaped downward pressure.

Harvesting colostrum

Harvesting colostrum is another term for hand-expressing in pregnancy. Towards the end of the third trimester (earlier for some women) you may already be leaking colostrum. Colostrum is liquid gold and is full of so much goodness for your little one. You can start harvesting colostrum from 37 weeks and it has many benefits for birth preparation.

- The act of nipple stimulation from the expressing can help to soften and ripen the cervix ready for birth.

- The sensation of hand-expressing colostrum can help mums-to-be get used to their breasts being stimulated in a very different way, which can take a while to adjust to.

- Once you have collected the colostrum in a sterilised pot, it can be collected into little syringes (you can get these from your midwife) and stored in the freezer. Take this with you when you go to the hospital or defrost when baby is born at home, and it can be used if for any reason baby isn't latching well or requires extra fluids. (To sterilise your pot, put it in a large saucepan. Cover with water, making sure there are no air bubbles. Boil rapidly for 5 minutes, then turn off and allow the water to cool down before removing.)

- If you don't need the colostrum after birth, keep it in the freezer (if you haven't defrosted it already). You can use it as a soothing liquid later down the line if baby has a sticky eye or a sore bottom. Defrost and drip a couple of drops into the eye, or wipe over nappy rash. It really is one of nature's cure-alls.

HOW TO HARVEST COLOSTRUM

It's important to make sure that you are well nourished, hydrated and comfy before expressing.

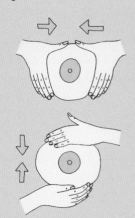

- Expose one breast and have your sterilised syringe and pot to hand. First, we need to prepare by stimulating the breast with gentle breast compressions. Place a hand on either side of the breast and compress and release (pulsing) for 1 minute. Next, place your hands on top and underneath the breast and repeat compressions for 1 minute.

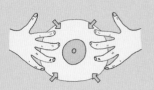

- To stimulate the oxytocin release and send the message to the brain to let the milk down, use the backs of your fingers to 'rake' from the outside edges of the breast to the edge of the areola (sort of dragging your fingers with a little pressure into the breast). Do this for 1 minute.

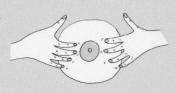

- Using the tips of the fingers, do what we call a 'pitter patter' massage all over the breast, like you are mimicking the pitter patter of rain. Think cats digging their claws into their mums for milk - it's that sort of thing, but not as hard.

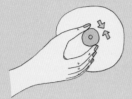

- Place your thumb at the top outer edge of the areola and the index finger at the bottom. Try and make sure they are lined up with each other, and make sure they are on the areola and not the nipple, otherwise you can make yourself sore (we are mimicking a baby's latch here).

- Using the thumb and index finger, press in towards your back, gently squeeze and then pull forwards, repeat in a rhythmic movement, again mimicking the sucking movement of a baby. After a few squeezes you should start to see little drops of colostrum coming out of the nipple. The colostrum will come out drop by drop, as it is thick and creamy. Watching a movie, or listening to a podcast is great to keep you distracted and stop you from getting bored. Change breasts once you notice the droplets have stopped or you start to feel uncomfortable.

- Once you have expressed from both breasts, use a syringe to collect the colostrum from your sterilised pot, label and pop it in the freezer. It will keep for 12 months. Defrost at room temperature and store in the fridge for 3 days. Do not re-freeze.

Please don't worry if you don't express much colostrum at the moment — remember, babies are way better at emptying the breasts than any hand or machine, and all breasts are different. Your colostrum will be in there, and it will come when baby is born.

157

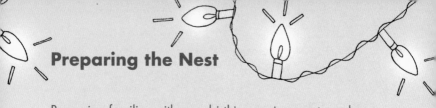

Preparing the Nest

Becoming familiar with your birthing environment can be very helpful for settling match-day nerves and keeping that adrenaline in check. Whether you are planning to birth at hospital or at home, it's good to familiarise yourself with what you will want your birthing environment to look like so that you can get everything ready.

If you are planning a hospital birth

- See if you can go for a tour of the ward – or at the very least just check out which part of the hospital you need to go to, so you aren't trying to find the labour ward while you're in actual labour!

- Familiarise yourself with the journey there. Will you drive or get a taxi, or will this depend on the time of day? Getting your head around all of this stuff before the big day will allow you to feel a little more at ease in the run-up to birth day.

- LED candles or fairy lights are great to take with you, so that you can create the twinkly low lighting that oxytocin likes in any hospital room.

- See our 'what to pack in your birth bag' checklist for some great ideas to enhance your birthing space (see pages 164–167).

If you are planning a home birth

We have both experienced home births from the perspective of birthing ourselves and in professional capacities, and know how calm it can be to labour and birth in your home environment. At a home birth, everything comes to you, and once your baby arrives your midwives will make sure you are all settled and well and will leave you to it, returning the following day to check in on your little family. In short, if all goes to plan, you get to remain undisturbed in your little birthing bubble and that can be an attractive option for many women.

- Start getting your birthing room ready. Which room will you be in? Think about where you will feel most cosy and at ease – that's probably the place to be.

- Will you hire a pool, or buy an inflatable one (they make great paddling pools after the event!)? If you are planning on using a birth pool, do test out the hose and tap connector before the big day. You'll be surprised how different all taps are, and let us tell you, filling up a birth pool by hand takes AGES!!!

- Think about lighting. Will you want low lighting? (Fairy lights and LED candles are great for this.)

- Allow yourself to nest – getting your home nice and clean and ready for you to hunker down and get to know your little one can help you to feel mentally calm. If you don't have time, are too tired or physically unable, ask a friend or family member to come and help you do a deep clean – or better still, get a cleaner in!

- Waterproof the rooms you've chosen by getting hold of tarpaulins or shower curtains and spreading them out on the carpet or over the bed or sofa, covered by clean towels and sheets for your comfort. Get a pile of old towels together for during and after the birth.

- Get hold of an anglepoise lamp or a powerful torch so that your midwife has good lighting when checking you down below following birth. They will need to see what they are doing clearly if you require stitches.

- Stock your cupboards and freezer with food and drink that you will enjoy during labour and following birth – and a packet of biscuits for the midwives to munch on with a cuppa always goes down well!

- Gather everything for your home birth together before the day arrives and put it all somewhere where you can find it all easily, so you don't have to cause yourself any stress when the day arrives.

- Prepare for a change in your home-birth plan if you need to transfer for some reason into the hospital. Have clothes, shoes and a birth bag for you and baby packed and ready just in case.

- Maybe buy a nice postnatal herbal bath blend ready for a healing bath once baby has arrived – it's great for sore perineums!

Visual wall

This is a lovely thing to do if visuals inspire you, whether you are planning on having a home birth or hospital birth, as we know that it can often help women feel calmer and more relaxed and able to stay at home for longer before transferring in.

If you're planning a home birth, choose one of the walls to stick up lots of lovely pictures. Think family photos that make you smile: maybe your scan pictures, any positive birthing affirmations you've seen, maybe you love the beach or forest and you can pop pictures up of those places to help yourself imagine you are there. Choose pictures that make you feel calm, free and happy – anything that will get that oxytocin going. If you are planning to birth in hospital, make a mood board to take with you.

We've been at lots of births where women have looked at the wall of pictures between surges and we can see the comfort and energy it can give them – we've also loved hearing about each picture and its meaning to the birthing mother.

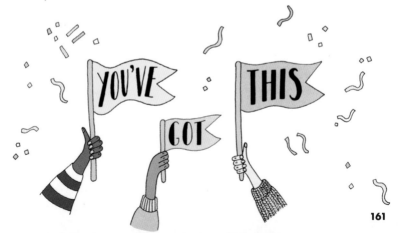

Food, glorious food

If you are planning a hospital birth, make sure you and your birthing partner both have your own snack bags as you will both need to eat. We've seen lots of birth partners stress-eat their way through a labour, and the last thing you want when you need it most is for there to be no snacks left. Some good labour snacks include:

- Biscuits (fig rolls are a firm fave for lots of our ladies)
- Chocolate raisins
- Little bite-sized chunks of fruit like chopped apples, mango, melon and satsuma – watery, sweet fruits are great for bursts of energy
- Protein is ideal for keeping your strength up if it's a long one – this can either be a protein shake, little bites of cooked egg or chicken, or a protein bar

Whether you plan to have your baby at home or at hospital, one thing is for sure: once they are out, you've both been checked, given the all-clear, the adrenaline has settled down and the oxytocin kicks in again, you'll suddenly feel HUNGRY!

We highly recommend packing a post-birth feast that you can tuck into as soon as you have been settled in your own bed or on a postnatal ward. Put some time and effort into this and really think about what you would love to sink your teeth into after a hard day's work!

groaning cake

There is an old English tradition for mothers to bake a cake during early labour called a 'Groaning Cake'. The smell of the baking was said to ease any pain and if a mother cracked the eggs her labour would be quick (it's worth a try!). There's no denying that a calm, therapeutic activity such as baking in early labour can be a good distraction (unless you can nap, then this would always be our first suggestion!). Baking smells definitely make us feel calm and cosy (good for the oxytocin), AND who doesn't like a cuppa and a bit of cake – either mid labour to keep your strength up, or once baby is born, as a celebration?! Traditionally, the cake was shared with families and friends once baby had arrived, to bring prosperity.

3 medium eggs
125ml vegetable oil,
  plus extra for greasing
120ml orange juice
100g molasses
  (or black treacle)
200g caster sugar

200g plain flour
2 teaspoons baking powder
1 teaspoon bicarbonate of soda
2 teaspoons ground cinnamon
1–2 teaspoons ground cloves
180g peeled and grated apples
1 teaspoon almond extract

Preheat the oven to 180°C/160°C fan. Beat the eggs in a large bowl and add the oil, orange juice, molasses and sugar. Sift the dry ingredients together into a separate medium bowl then stir in the grated apples. Add the dry ingredients to the wet, mix well and stir through the almond extract. Tip into a greased 2lb loaf tin and bake in the oven for 35–40 minutes.

Remove from the oven and leave to cool in the tin for 15 minutes, then transfer to a wire rack to cool. It will keep for 5 days in an airtight container, if it lasts that long!

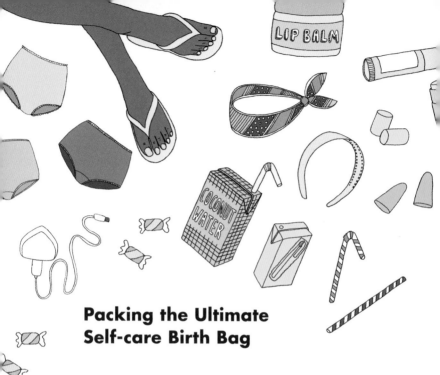

Packing the Ultimate Self-care Birth Bag

There are hundreds of sites online that talk you through what to pack for baby, but here we want to focus on you, and what to pack in your birth bag to keep you as comfortable as possible throughout birth and once babe arrives. Whether you are planning to birth at home or at hospital, it is a good idea to pack a birth bag. If you do stay at home, you will then have everything you need in one place, and if for any reason you do need to transfer to hospital, your bag will be ready to go.

This list has been compiled over many years, and the result of seeing many a birth bag along the way. You don't have to pack everything that is on it, but have a good look through and choose the items that you feel you would like to have with you.

❑ Your notes and your birth plan.

❑ Coconut water – with naturally occurring electrolytes, this is the perfect rehydrating drink.

❑ Frozen bottles of water – pop a couple of water bottles in the freezer and grab them on your way out – they will melt gradually, leaving you with ice-cold water.

❑ A flask of ice cubes – some ladies love to crunch ice in labour.

❑ Snacks (see page 162).

❑ Ginger chews – great for sickness and a hit of sugar. These can be purchased from health food shops.

❑ Date syrup. This is perfect if you don't fancy eating but need to keep your energy up and get a sugar fix. You can have it straight off the spoon or in tea.

❑ Herbal tea bags.

❑ Reusable straws, to help keep that jaw nice and loose.

❑ Moisturiser.

❑ Lip balm – lips get very dry in labour.

❑ Natural nipple cream.

❑ Nice toiletries for that awesome postnatal shower.

❑ Refreshing face spritz.

- ❏ Hair ties, clips, headband and hairbrush.

- ❏ Essential oils, massage oil and a flannel.

- ❏ Oversized T-shirt and light dressing gown, plus some soft, cosy PJs and soft, loose clothes to travel home in.

- ❏ Bikini if you are planning a water birth (only if you'd like to wear one – you don't have to!).

- ❏ Fluffy socks and some cosy slippers (in case of epidural – you will want to keep your feet warm to stop you feeling chilly and shaky).

- ❏ Glorious granny pants – comfort is paramount.

- ❏ BIG maternity pads.

- ❏ Glasses – if you wear contact lenses, make sure you remember to pack your glasses, too.

- ❏ A well-fitting feeding bra – you want something soft and supportive, for when the milk comes and your breasts can be very tender.

- ❏ Eye mask and ear plugs to help you rest in labour and postnatally.

- ❏ Blanket or big shawl – great to get cosy, if you want a nap.

- ❏ A couple of pillows from home.

❑ Your handwritten favourite affirmations (see page 95).

❑ Phone and extra-long phone charging cable, so that you can have your phone in bed, plugged in, without having to get up.

❑ Earphones – to listen to any hypnobirthing tracks or guided meditations you may have or just drown out the hospital noise and listen to music.

❑ LED candles or fairy lights, if you'd like to keep the lighting low.

❑ Hand-held fan – so great when you are feeling hot and flustered.

❑ Bluetooth speaker for your birth tunes.

❑ Your birth letters – see cultural traditions on page 148.

❑ Hot water bottle in case of any post-birth aches and pains – also great to use in labour.

Once you have packed your bag, we highly recommend tipping it all out on the bed and getting your birth partner to repack it (with your assistance, of course). This way they will familiarise themselves with what's in your bag and know where it all is.

Fourth Trimester Plan

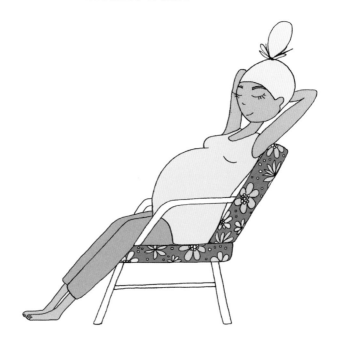

During pregnancy we often spend time looking after ourselves really well, then once our baby arrives, life with a newborn takes over and we may feel that layer of support and nurture start to fizzle out or get redirected towards the baby.

The great news is that it really doesn't have to be that way and it only takes a little planning and preparation before your baby arrives to start the wheel of postnatal self-care turning to ensure that you bring those lovely nurturing elements into the fold. The best time to arrange the details for a slow and self-care-centric postnatal period is when you are still pregnant so that your support network can be utilised from the moment your baby arrives.

Our tips for writing a game-changing fourth trimester plan

Make a plan for at least the first six weeks post birth in two sections:

(1) self-care (what you can do for yourself) and (2) community care (what support can you bring in from friends and family or hired help).

1. Postnatal slow-down
Prepare for one week in bed and one on the sofa: we are really referring here to resting as much as is possible in those first couple of weeks (with gentle physical mobilisation throughout). If you find the walls are closing in, do get some fresh air or take a gentle walk outside but don't overdo it or you will likely feel your energy plummet again very quickly!

2. Don't mistake adrenaline for energy
Over the years many women have said to us that they thought they had the energy to take on anything after birth only to find that after a few days the combination of post-birth fatigue and the swift drop of pregnancy hormones left them feeling completely depleted of energy and on their knees with exhaustion. Listen to your body, rest as much as possible and remember that with energy, what goes up must come down.

3. Make your postnatal nest
When possible, encourage a calm and nurturing environment at home. You and your baby are both making this huge transition together. In order to encourage oxytocin release, have plenty of skin-to-skin (can be a cuddle, not just for feeding), let them hear your heartbeat and voice, and take in your family's smell.

4. Check in on yourself

Plan to keep an eye on your physical and mental health in the days, weeks and months that follow birth. Remember to talk to your partner, midwife, health visitor or GP if you are feeling overly sore or uncomfortable, or if you are worried at all that you are experiencing regular bouts of low, anxious or vacant mood. They will be able to help and support your physical and mental wellbeing.

5. Avoid hosting!

When planning who will come to see you and meet the baby, remember you will be healing, your baby will be transitioning from womb to world and you and your partner will be adapting to being parents. If friends and family are coming over for a cuddle with the new baby and ask if they can help in anyway, don't be afraid to let them play their part in lightening the load. Having somebody empty the dishwasher, hang out a load of washing, pick up some essentials from the shops or entertain your other children for you can be so helpful.

6. Celebratory feast

In many cultures, food is a hugely important part of postnatal healing. Think about the food you love to eat and fill your freezer to the brim with your favourite nosh before your baby makes an appearance.

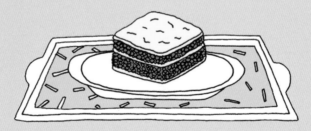

The Waiting Game!

Lots of women worry about going overdue, but the irony is that worry can be the very thing that sometimes delays labour. Our birth hormone, oxytocin, is released when we are relaxed and feel safe. Too much adrenaline, our stress hormone, stops the production of oxytocin, so in theory can stop us going into labour.

Our first suggestion, then, would be to stop worrying! Easier said than done, right? How about reminding yourself that our estimated due date is just that, an estimation, and actually very few women give birth on their due date!

Just remember that your healthcare team will be keeping a close eye on you, they will get you to monitor baby's movements, and your midwife will do all the necessary checks to make sure that you and baby are okay.

You may be feeling well and truly fed up by now. You may have swollen feet, sleep might be tricky and you just may have had enough with well-wishers texting you asking if there's 'any news' (believe us we know, we've been there), as if you'd have the baby and forget to tell people!

Turn off your phone and think about what will make you feel better – a day in bed watching box-sets with the odd trip back and forth to the loo and the kitchen, maybe a nice swim so you can enjoy feeling weightless in the water, or maybe some good belly laughs over lunch with your best mate. Just remember that you won't be pregnant forever (we know it can feel that way) and that the best thing you can do for yourself right now is be as kind to yourself as possible, and do whatever fills your cup up.

While there is no eject button, there are some 'natural methods' that you can try to nudge baby into playing ball and coming out to play!

Although it is definitely worth trying some of the below, don't get too hung up on trying everything to get labour going. We see women who are so stressed about getting labour started, they are almost certainly not going to go into labour because their stress hormones are too high. If your body is taking its own sweet time, you may be offered a medical induction and you can discuss the pros and cons with your midwife and come up with a care plan that you are both happy with.

Harvesting colostrum

Hand-expressing colostrum (see pages 155–157) is effectively nipple stimulation, which is known to soften the cervix, which may help the body to go into labour.

Sex

We know it can feel like an impossible feat when you are at full term and you have a sizeable bump, but if you can find a comfortable position, sex may boost oxytocin levels (see pages 106–109 for more on sex in pregnancy).

Bodywork

Any treatments that encourage you to relax and lower your stress hormones are going to help your body get the right balance of hormones for birth to begin. Acupuncture, reflexology and massage therapy have the added benefit of working on acupressure and reflex points known to stimulate the cervix – this can sometimes nudge the body into labour. Gentle exercise can also give you a lovely hit of happy hormones and calm adrenaline.

Homeopathy

Some homeopathic remedies are thought to help bring labour on, but always visit a qualified homeopath so you are using the remedies as safely as possible.

Some things you might like to include in your diet

6 dates a day!
Research suggests that dates have an oxytocin-like effect on the body, leading to increased sensitivity in the uterus. Eating 6 dates a day from thirty-six weeks is said to help to ripen the cervix and result in a quicker dilation. Worth a try, right! High in fibre, potassium, magnesium, folate and vitamin K, they also contain lots of nutrients a mum-to-be needs. Win win! If you can't face scoffing that many dates a day, try adding them to a smoothie.

Raspberry leaf tea
You can start drinking one cup of raspberry leaf tea a day from thirty-two weeks, upping to two cups from thirty-six weeks onwards, to help tonify the uterus ready for birth. Please do not drink this tea in the first trimester, and if you notice your Braxton Hicks increase after thirty-two weeks, stop drinking the tea and start again from thirty-seven weeks – some people may be more sensitive to the tea's effects than others.

Pineapple
Pineapple contains an enzyme called bromelain that is said to soften the cervix, which can help the body prepare for birth. You would need to eat fresh pineapple and LOTS of it to trigger labour, but adding pineapple to your daily diet may help stimulate the softening process preparing the cervix for birth.

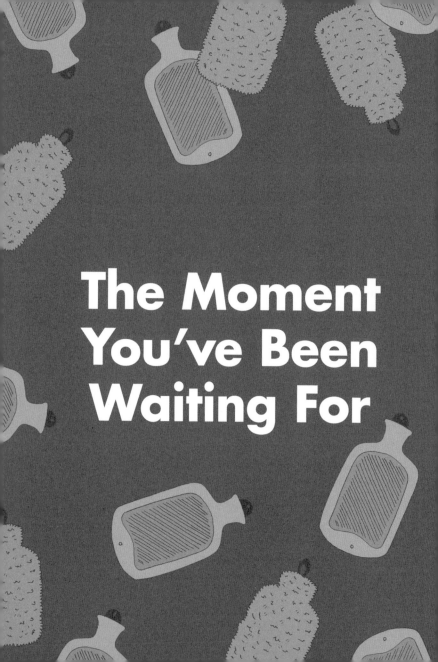

The Moment You've Been Waiting For

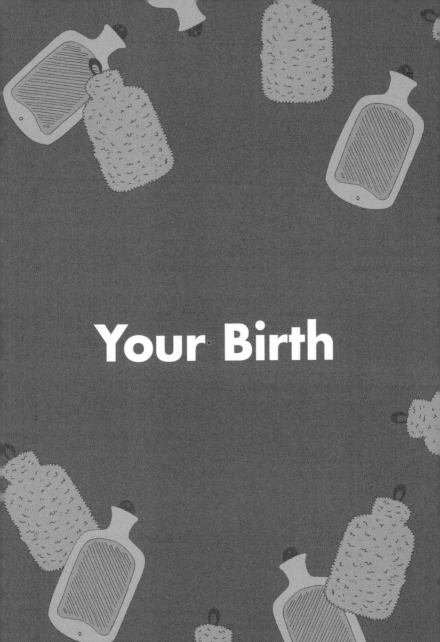

Your Birth

You are finally here: the moment you have been waiting for! It is difficult to put into words how you feel when you realise that you are about to meet your baby for the first time. Often the surge of birthing hormones is accompanied by a whole array of emotions. We can feel so excited and hugely fearful all at the same time, and this can leave us feeling a little frazzled.

Once again, we want to remind you that the only thing you need to worry about right now is keeping that oxytocin nice and high. Your body and your baby know how to do the rest, and your hugely important job is to stop adrenaline getting in their way, by keeping yourself as mentally calm and physically relaxed as you can.

We want to remind you at this point that when it comes to birthing, perfection is not what we are striving for. Birth is one of the most unpredictable things, and often the twists and turns our birth journey takes are out of our control. The best we can do is to remain calm and flexible, and to allow birth to unfold as it needs. There is no perfect birth, but there are beautiful births, there are amazing birth teams and there can be many perfect moments during this life-changing experience.

Remember, you have prepared your mind and body for this final event and you are as ready as you can be, so be gentle with yourself and trust in the process.

Lean on your birth team any time you feel the need, and remember you are not alone. All over the world right now there are thousands of women birthing their babies alongside you.

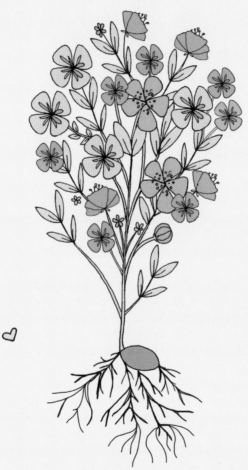

The Perfect Cocktail: Birth Hormones

When it comes to birthing, your hormones play an essential role. It is so important to truly understand how they can help or hinder the birthing process so you can work with your birthing body as effectively as possible.

Oxytocin

Aptly nicknamed the love hormone, oxytocin is released during sex, light and gentle touching, breastfeeding and birth. Think of it like a net that swoops in and wraps itself around the fibres of your body, rhythmically squeezing and releasing. Encouraging our love hormone to soar is vital in order to have effective, strong contractions because it travels through your blood flow into the fibres of your uterus and squeezes, thus creating a shortening of the muscle fibres, and hey presto, you have a contraction! If you have an induction or need help to regulate your contractions then you will be given a syntocinon drip, which is a synthetic version of your naturally occurring oxytocin.

Oxytocin is known to be a shy hormone that thrives when we feel unobserved, safe, loved, protected and calm. The need to find a quiet calm space when birthing is primal. Just like a cat will often choose to birth her kittens at the back of the garden shed, we have seen many birthing women over the years drawn towards a cosy corner of their home or hospital room where they can labour and birth feeling safer and less observed. One woman comes to mind, who tried to climb into her warm, cosy airing cupboard during a home birth. Following birth, she said that she was drawn to it as it felt like it would be safe and contained in there.

Creating a low-lit, comfortable nest for yourself is a wonderful way to help your oxytocin levels thrive, which in turn can have a very positive effect on your birthing body (revisit our section on making your nest on pages 158–160).

Nipple and clitoral stimulation, by yourself or your partner, can help release a surge of oxytocin, which can be helpful if contractions are slowing down or becoming irregular. There have been many times over the years when we have left couples for a little while to try to get things going again in private. Leaving you alone to have an oxytocin-releasing massage (see pages 182–183) or a canoodle, unobserved, can be a very effective way to get the body calm and relaxed again and release a lovely dose of oxytocin into your system.

You can also use a few drops of clary sage essential oil, sometimes referred to as nature's syntocinon for its ability to promote rhythmic contractions. Try a few drops on a paper fan or a flannel and hold it in front of your nose and mouth while practising the 3 Flamingos breath on page 26. (Important: do not use clary sage before thirty-seven weeks.)

Endorphins

Another key ingredient for our comfort and wellbeing during labour and birth are endorphins. These magical little naturally occurring chemicals are sometimes referred to as pleasure or happiness hormones. They are cleverly produced when your body faces strong physical sensations and have a pain-relieving and calming effect on us. In a similar way to opiates, endorphins steadily build up in your system as your labour and birth progresses, interacting with pain receptors in your brain and helping to take the edge off, reduce your discomfort and make you feel a natural kind of high.

Adrenaline

Sometimes adrenaline, our 'fight or flight' hormone, shows up to our birth party uninvited. As the hormone that is focused on protecting us and ensuring our survival, it likes to check in and make sure we are safe. The problem is that if left to thrive, adrenaline can have a detrimental effect on our birthing mind and body, pressing pause on the role of oxytocin and slowing down labour in order to protect you.

Apart from making you feel light-headed and sweaty, with a racing heart, adrenaline can also detract all-important blood flow and oxygen away from the uterus and into your hands and feet just in case you have to leg it away from danger or physically fight yourself out of harm's way.

The trick is to be responsive to your birthing mind and body. If you feel adrenaline bubbling away inside, counterbalance it and soothe yourself by promoting feelings of calm and control. You can have a huge impact on your hormones so remember to return to your breathwork, light touch massage, essential oils, resting, positive affirmations, relaxation scripts and lowering the lights where possible so you can get your oxytocin and endorphins flowing again.

TOP FIVE WAYS TO BOOST YOUR HAPPY HORMONE

1. **EAT YOUR FAVOURITE FOOD.** You may not feel like a big meal during labour, but a little of the food that brings you pleasure can help you release a surge of mood-boosting endorphins. Foods that have earned a reputation for being linked with our happy hormones are dark chocolate, strawberries, chilli (go easy), nuts and seeds (especially brazil nuts), oranges, eggs and bananas.

2. **LAUGH.** The more you giggle your way through your contractions, the more your endorphins will thrive! Choose a box-set that is going to make you LOL your way through early labour and keep you as comfortable and calm as possible, saving that all-important energy for later on, when you will need it the most.

3. **MUSIC.** We always suggest you make at least two playlists for labour and birth. One filled with music to anchor you in a calm, relaxed headspace, and one that bangs out the upbeat tunes and gets you swaying your birthing hips to the beat, giving you a lovely surge in energy.

4. **LAVENDER.** Get out your lavender flannel (see page 198) and waft that birthing ninja all around your bad self! Research has found that lavender naturally sedates and eases discomfort by encouraging a lovely endorphin release.

5. **LET'S GET IT ON.** Just like oxytocin, endorphins are released when we enjoy a loving smooch-fest with our partners. Spend some time in early labour having some skin-to-skin time together to get those warm and fuzzy vibes going.

Oxytocin-releasing light touch massage

By offering soothing touch to a pregnant or birthing woman we can provide much comfort and help keep those birthing hormones flowing. It is so simple and easy to do! Begin light touch massage by encouraging mum-to-be to close her eyes, relax and drop her shoulders, and become controlled and intentional in regards to slowing down her breath.

Neck and head
Instructions for your partner:

1. Sit behind mum-to-be and start with the upper side of your fingertips at the base of the neck (where the neck meets the back).

2. Slowly trace your fingers up the neck, over the hair and to the top of the head.

3. Keep your fingers in place there for a moment and apply gentle pressure with splayed fingertips.

4. Trace the underside of your fingertips back down over the hair, down the neck and back to your starting position.

5. Repeat for at least 5 minutes.

Back

Instructions for your partner:

1. Start sitting or kneeling behind mum to-be so that her back is facing you completely exposed, or with a light, fitted top so that she can feel your touch.

2. Place the palms of your hands either side of the spine, flat against her sacrum (the flat, hard area at the bottom of the back) and apply controlled medium pressure with whole hands.

3. Use the palms of your hands to walk (literally like feet walking one at a time) up the back gently, always keeping your hands either side of the spine.

4. Once you reach the top of the back, move your hands up and over, softly squeezing her shoulders, either side of the base of the neck, and remind her to relax them down and release any trapped tension.

5. Use the underside of the fingertips to trace back down the back in a wavy motion.

6. Repeat for at least 5 minutes.

PLEASE NOTE:
You can adjust this massage if mum-to-be is in the birthing pool, leaning forwards, so that you stand, sit or kneel in front of her. Start in the same position at the base of the neck, this time using the underside of your fingertips and travelling the light touch towards yourself and to the top of her head, then continue the sequence in reverse, back to the base of the neck, but this time away from yourself.

Birth Part 1 – The Latent Phase

Your baby's eviction notice has finally been served and things are starting to happen. The 'latent phase' is usually the longest stage of your labour, and in some cases it can last several days before established (active) labour begins.

This phase can range from feeling lower abdominal tightenings or lower backache that is mild and irregular, to powerful sensations that begin to form a rhythmic and established pattern.

Labour can often start in the night time while we are asleep because we are relaxed, our adrenaline is low and our birthing hormones, oxytocin and endorphins can build up effectively, undisturbed. When everything begins happening you may initially experience a surge in adrenaline. It is completely natural to have this response, after all, you are about to go through your birthing journey that will result in you finally meeting your baby.

We always tell the couples we work with that what you do at this important time can set the tone for your whole birthing experience. You can start by really paying attention to helping yourself stay as calm as possible during early labour by following our tips opposite.

A balance between movement and rest is key here. If labour starts during the night, we urge you to try and go back to sleep, or at least rest for as long as you can. Once day breaks, or when you feel the need to be upright, try some gentle movement to jiggle that baby down into the pelvis.

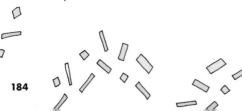

Top tips for the Latent Phase

- **Rest.** It may be hard to get some solid shut-eye once things get started, but do try to conserve your precious energy, dozing where possible or resting by snuggling up with your pillows and blankets on the sofa.

- **Keep lighting low.** Low lighting can encourage a relaxed and calm response in our brain. Oxytocin is released in softer light, especially when you're surrounded by warm colours such as pinks and reds

> **LABOUR LIGHTING**
> Himalayan salt lamps are great to help create the perfect hue and low-lit, calm ambience for the birth setting. It can also be lovely for creating a softly lit atmosphere during night feeds once baby arrives.

- **Get cosy and comfortable.** You are likely to be more aware of sensory stimulation during labour, so make sure your clothes are soft, comfortable and non-restrictive.

- **Get the right pong in the air.** Grab your favourite sumptuous body lotions, scented candles or essential oils.

- **Breathe.** If you feel that your adrenaline is getting the better of you, always return to the 'opening breath' (see page 133). This can help you soothe and comfort yourself back to feeling calm and in control.

- **Line up some distractions.** In the early stages you may find that distracting yourself from those irregular tightenings can actually help the time go faster. It can be worth lining up hypnobirthing tracks, favourite podcasts, TV shows and music playlists to help distract the mind and stop you from overthinking.

- **Take a walk on the wild side.** If you know that being in nature will refresh and calm your mind and body then head out (taking your maternity notes with you) and take a gentle walk, being mindful of not overstimulating your adrenal responses (and don't wander too far!).

- **Pace yourself.** Be kind to yourself and your body and allow it to take the time it needs. Remember, labour can take a while, and you wouldn't start a marathon with a sprint, would you! Take it slow, potter, and try to keep that adrenaline low. Slow and steady wins the race.

- **Choose a change of scenery.** The old adage 'a change is as good as a rest' really is true. If labour feels like it's been going for a while and you are feeling flat, try changing rooms for a bit of a lift.

- **Fuel yourself.** Do keep eating and drinking. You may not feel like eating much in the later stages, so try and eat now while you can. If you are feeling queasy, stick to bland foods, eating little and often, and focus on really keeping your fluids up. Take little sips regularly – no gulping or you'll feel sick.

- **Take a dip.** A nice soak will help to relax your muscles and can ease the discomfort of the cramping because warm water helps us to release endorphins.

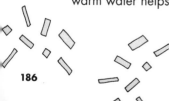

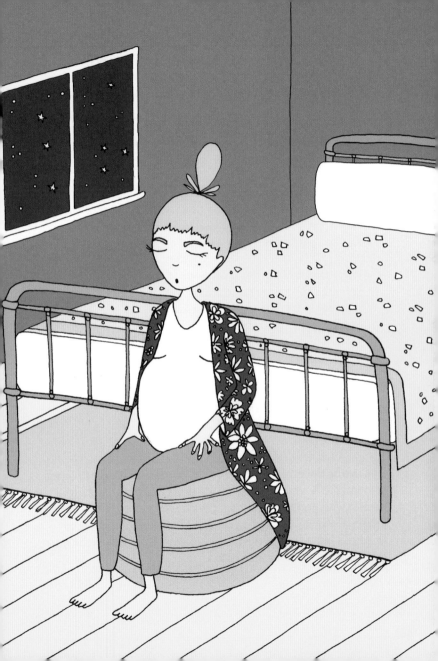

- **Wiggle those hips.** Moving your hips can really help baby to wiggle down into the pelvis, so sway, pretend to hula, draw figures of eight with your hips and try walking up and down the stairs sideways (holding onto the banister to steady yourself) or have a gentle bounce on your birthing ball. These are all fab ways to release and open the hips to help baby's descent.

- **Use a TENS machine.** If you have one, use it now to help ease discomfort. Even if you don't want to use it at this stage, get your partner to practise putting it on before labour progresses.

- **Hot water bottle.** Place the heat on the lower back to ease back cramps, or between your legs to ease pelvic pain. Don't use it on your bump, and remember not to have it too hot (too much heat can make you feel a bit light-headed or a bit unwell) and make sure it is covered so you don't burn yourself. If you are overly hot, try putting the hot water bottle in the freezer and using it as an ice pack instead, to keep you cool.

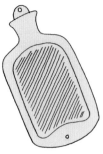

This is a really exciting time, so you might be tempted to send a round robin message that things are cracking on but be careful who you tell! If labour takes a while to progress you may not want to be fielding people's texts and enquiries as to what's happening, which can happen when well-meaning friends or family get over-excited.

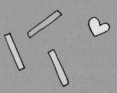

'Birth is such a lesson in letting go of expectations and following your instinct. The one thing my rational brain told me I didn't want this time around (my daughter's presence at my home birth) turned out to be the very thing I needed to birth her little brother. I couldn't have done it without her little hands sploshing water on my back and her cheeky smile helping me through.'

ANOUSHKA, MUM OF TWO

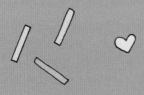

WORD TO THE BIRTH PARTNER

Your birth partner will be a very important person during your labour. Your midwife and doctors will be skilled and experienced at building a rapport with you quickly, but it is highly possible that you may not have met them before. However, your birth partner will know you so well already and can jump straight in to looking after you with pre-existing trust. Our top tips for birth partners:

DOCTOR OXYTOCIN

Think of your main role throughout birthing to be the one who keeps oxytocin (the love hormone) sky high! Help mum-to-be build that nest and create that cosy, gentle environment where birthing hormones can thrive and adrenaline will be kept at bay. Keep the lighting low and relaxing and provide comfort through touch (see light touch massage on pages 182-183). Offer gentle verbal encouragement and oodles of TLC.

DRINK UP

Dehydration can lead to a longer, more painful labour and isn't ideal for baby either. So make sure mum-to-be is well hydrated with regular sips of water, or better still coconut water that has naturally occurring electrolytes present.

A WEE REMINDER

Encourage her to go for a wee every couple of hours (unless she is still able to sleep and tightenings remain very irregular). As labour progresses we don't want a full bladder to hold that baby back. If she is not needing a wee every two hours then up the sips of fluid. The rule of thumb is if she feels thirsty then it's a sign she is already getting dehydrated.

KEEP HER FED

Eating little and often is very important throughout labour so that energy reserves are kept high. This can be easier said than done if she is feeling nauseous or has lost her appetite. Keep food and snacks available so that she can have a nibble if she feels up to it. Simple snacks to scoff are a piece of fruit such as a banana, energy balls (see page 34) a granola bar, a slice of toast, a few squares of chocolate, or jelly sweets. There should be plenty of snacks in your bag! (See page 164.)

UPRIGHT NOT UPTIGHT

Encourage her to stay upright and potter around gently or sit on a birthing ball and slowly rock back and forth or side to side. It helps keep things moving and supports baby into the most ideal position for birthing. However, if it is night time and you are both able to sleep, take full advantage of this rest time.

TAKE CONTROL

Sort out the logistics so that mum-to-be is not burdened with any unnecessary worries, such as care for other kids or pets (including making lists and packing bags for anyone looking after them), cancelling appointments or social events (i.e. dinner with the neighbours or your boiler being serviced), organising transport to hospital if relevant, and gathering the birth bags, maternity notes and any frozen colostrum.

KEEP CALM

Remind yourself and mum-to-be to conserve energy during early labour and do all you can to help her stay calm. If you are feeling your own adrenaline building, employ tactics that will help you feel refreshed: rest, take a shower, practise mindfulness, get some fresh air, try deep, slow breathing.

STAY POSITIVE

Steer clear of negative language like 'is it painful?' or 'this is hard'. Instead, encourage her with positive words. If she says, 'I can't do this,' tell her 'you are doing it' and 'you are doing so well.' Instead of counting contractions to come, celebrate their passing with 'that's another one gone!' or 'that was a good one.' Read some affirmations, see page 95).

LOOK AFTER YOURSELF

Keep rested, hydrated and fed so you can be present and alert for mum-to-be as labour progresses. We have had birth partners faint during birth because they were dehydrated and exhausted.

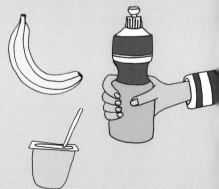

Waterworks

Often, women expect that the first sign of labour will be a gush of their waters breaking (the releasing of their amniotic fluid) as that tends to be what we see on TV. In reality this happens in less than 10 per cent of labours. If you think your waters have broken, pop a maternity pad on and give your maternity unit a call. It may be that your baby is using your bladder as a trampoline and a little bit of wee has escaped. It's tricky to confirm until your midwife sees you in person, puts a speculum in your vagina and takes a look for evidence of leaking water and a sample to see whether there is amniotic fluid present. If it is your waters that are being released, it is likely:

- To be clear or pinky coloured (or occasionally green, see below).
- Not to smell of wee, but will smell sweet and yeasty.
- That you will have no control over them.
- That they will keep trickling out as your baby moves.

If it is confirmed that your waters have indeed broken, but contractions have not started, your midwife will send you home to await events for 6–12 hours (depending on your hospital policy). You will be encouraged to go back in after this time to be assessed and an induction may be advised, as waters breaking means that there is now a throughway to your baby, which increases the risk of infection.

> **PLEASE NOTE:** If the water is a greenish colour it can be an indication that your baby has done a poo, and the midwife will want to know about it and will get you to head in to the hospital promptly to monitor the baby more closely and make sure they are happy in there.

Call the midwife

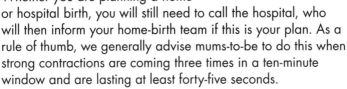

Once labour progresses you will need to call the hospital and let them know what's happening. Whether you are planning a home or hospital birth, you will still need to call the hospital, who will then inform your home-birth team if this is your plan. As a rule of thumb, we generally advise mums-to-be to do this when strong contractions are coming three times in a ten-minute window and are lasting at least forty-five seconds.

REMEMBER: 3–10–45!

If you are birthing at home, your birth team will call in to check on you and will make a plan as to whether they stay or leave you for a little while longer.

If you are planning a hospital birth, you will pop along to triage to be assessed. Packing up and 'heading in' can feel quite daunting and overwhelming for your senses, especially if you are feeling nested and comfortable in your home environment, but there are ways to manage the journey in, while protecting your oxytocin levels (see over the page).

TOP TIPS FOR HEADING IN

- **Don't forget your maternity notes!!!!** We would underline this twice if we could.

- Have your birth bags packed and ready to go so you can leave it to your birthing partner to gather them together and load them up.

- Wear comfortable clothing that requires minimal effort and will not aggravate you or restrict your movement. Make sure you are warm enough, with a cosy cardigan or jumper so that you do not need to fuss about any external physical sensations and you can concentrate on remaining in control during your contractions on the way in.

- Keep your sensory load to a minimum, especially if you are stepping out of a quiet, calm, gently lit environment. The last thing we want is for your oxytocin to get spooked and run for the hills. You can do this by taking a warm, cosy blanket to wrap around yourself in the car, wearing headphones and playing calming music or hypnobirthing scripts, and taking an eye mask or sunglasses if it's bright and busy.

- Let your birth partner manage the logistics of how you will get to the birth unit. Make sure they have planned in advance whether they will drive you or you will head in together by taxi.

- Take your lavender flannel (see page 198) with you and focus on your breathwork the whole way in.

- Take a large incontinence pad with you (a square disposable, absorbent pad available at pharmacies and online) and sit on it with an old towel on top. These are ideal for if your waters have broken already and have the potential to leak through your maternity pad, or if your waters break en route. Either way, it's just another thing you don't have to worry about.

Ways to set the scene

Once you are taken to your designated room it's time to recreate that nest again. You may find your contractions have lost a little bit of their welly as adrenaline has been more prevalent during the home-to-hospital transfer and you have come in contact with the new faces of the staff. Worry not! You can employ all your lovely adrenaline-calming breathing techniques and oxytocin- and endorphin-releasing light touch massage to get your birthing mojo in full flow again.

Unless there is a good reason to be on that hospital bed, push it out of the way or turn it into a chair (the beds usually have clever mechanisms which enable them to take on an armchair shape). Ask the midwife to bring in the birthing ball and bean bags, unpack your own pillows and blankets that you may have brought in from home to make your space feel safe, cosy and appealing. This set-up will encourage you to adopt a UFO (Upright, Forward, Open) position, which is perfect for your birthing body as it works with gravity and makes the best space possible in your pelvis for baby's birth.

- Turn those lights down low and get out your LED candles or fairy lights to create a gentle glow in your birth space.

- Kick off your shoes and any restrictive clothing and get into your birthing garb. Cosy joggers, loose-fitting T-shirt, nightie, tankini top and bikini bottoms for a water birth or fully naked if that feels best. Whatever ensemble you choose, make sure your clothes are not causing you any sensory distraction and you are as comfy as possible.

- Ask the midwives if they have any essential oils you can make use of (often labour wards will keep a small selection). Or use oils that you have brought with you.

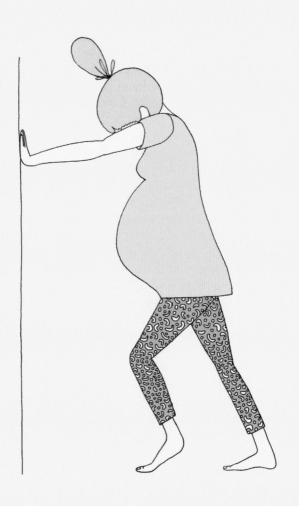

Birth Part 2 – Established Labour

You are likely to get to a point during your early labour when things start hotting up and you just feel like there has been a change in sensation. At this stage you may feel like strong contractions are washing over you with purpose. They are more intense and powerful and that is normal and will be encouraging your cervix to open. Take them one at a time and employ everything we have spoken about in preparation to keep that wind in your sails.

During this time you will need oodles of support and comfort from your birth partner to keep you going. Your main job here is to surrender to birth and allow yourself to let go and be supported by those around you.

TOP TIPS FOR ESTABLISHED LABOUR

PAIN-RELIEVING PONGS
Essential oils can be really helpful when it comes to easing aches and pains. Black pepper, lavender and clary sage are our favourites for birth. Remember that your sense of smell is very strong during labour, so place 4 drops of oil on a tissue or a paper fan (this can just be a piece of A4 paper, folded into a concertina shape) so that you can control the usage, and remove the oils completely if you find that they are too strong for you.

LAVENDER FLANNEL
The ninja in the birth room!
1. Wet a flannel with cold water. Add 4 drops of lavender essential oil.
2. Squeeze out the excess water and fold the flannel over so that the drops of oil are inside the fold and won't directly touch the skin.
3. Let mum-to-be hold the flannel, or place it on her forehead to cool her down if she is hot.
4. Encourage mum-to-be to breathe deeply into the flannel with each surge.
5. When the flannel loses its strength or gets too warm, refresh it with water and a few more drops of lavender oil.

A QUICK CHANGE-UP
It is not uncommon for a labouring mum to get really attached to one position during labour, but it is important to move frequently to help jiggle baby down the pelvic canal and to keep the body soft and open. We advise weeing every 2 hours during labour to ensure a full bladder isn't impinging baby's pathway. Use this as a chance to change position.

GO BACK TO THE BREATH
We really believe there is no better way to reset if you start to feel that adrenaline bubbling. This is the time to reap the fruits of your labour (pardon the pun) and use all of the breathing exercises you have practised during your pregnancy. Ask your partner to read you the relaxation script on page 127 as you focus on breathing through each surge.

EYES ON THE PRIZE!
When things aren't progressing as quickly as we'd like, or we are tired and uncomfortable, it can be easy to lose sight of the end. Keep your eyes on the prize: every time you hit a wall, imagine that first snuggle to keep you going!

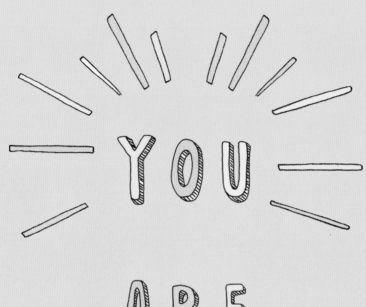

YOU

ARE

AWESOME

PAIN RELIEF IN HOSPITAL

If you decide that you need further support to cope
with the strong sensations of labour, there will be
a number of pain-relieving options available in most
hospitals. We are not going to go through the hows and
whys of each pain relief method here as you can find
that info in birth manuals or via your midwife. What we
do want to share with you is how to care for yourself
well if you do go for any of the mentioned options.

PETHIDINE OR DIAMORPHINE

Most commonly used if you experience a very
long latent phase. If you do opt for pethidine
or diamorphine:

- Lie down on your
  left side and get
  as comfortable as
  possible.

- Get some peppermint
  essential oil ready on
  a paper towel or cool
  wet flannel to place
  on your forehead as
  you may feel nauseous
  (though the injection
  will be given with
  an anti-sickness
  medication).

- Take sips of water
  with the help of your
  midwife or partner,
  to help you stay
  hydrated.

- If you feel sick,
  use our sickness
  and nausea-relieving
  breathing technique
  on page 26.

- Close your eyes
  and shut off any
  unnecessary outside
  sensory stimulation,
  and rest.

GAS AND AIR (ENTONOX)

Can be used at home or at hospital from around 5cm
dilated. When using gas and air:

- You may find it helpful to close your eyes and have
  the midwife or your birthing partner help balance
  you if you start to feel dizzy or woozy.

- Use lavender and peppermint essential oil on a wet flannel or a paper fan to help soothe any nausea (see page 198).

- Sip water in between contractions as gas and air can be quite dehydrating.

- Use a moisturising lip balm, as you can get very dry, cracked lips from using it over a number of hours.

EPIDURAL ....

Known to be a full pain-receptor block administered at hospital. If you opt for an epidural:

- Get into a comfy position before the cannula and wires are attached to your arm (even with a 'mobile epidural' you will be less mobile). This may mean taking your bra off or changing into a different loose-fitting T-shirt or hospital gown. You can do it later on, but it will just be a little more tricky.

- Refrain from using essential oils that lower your blood pressure, such as ylang ylang, lavender, frankincense or clary sage, as the fluids that are going into your arm are trying to prevent you from getting low blood pressure.

- Pop on a pair of cosy socks or wrap a soft blanket around you if you start to shiver and tremble. This can be a side effect of the medication and is nothing to worry about; your midwife will be with you and will help keep you as comfortable as possible.

- Make the most of the rest and sleep if you can, as you will still need your energy to push your baby out!

Transition

From pulling to pushing

So once again your brilliant body shifts a gear and moves to the next phase. At this point the sensations you are experiencing can change, and you may feel more intense pressure and stretching as your baby starts to move down a little further. Some women will move from one stage of labour to the next barely noticing the change, but for many women transition can be an emotionally trying time. If this occurs during your labour, know that this is completely normal; your midwife will have supported women through transition time and time again, and you will pass through these feelings.

As you pass through transition and into the second stage, where you will birth your baby, your focus will change again and the sensations of birth will alter as your uterus contracts with the strength to encourage your baby down. You will often find you have no choice but to let go and allow those involuntary pushes lead you.

Five things to do to support a mum-to-be in transition

- She may well say something like 'I can't do it,' 'I want to have an epidural,' or 'give me a caesarean section,' at this point. The sensations of transition can feel too big, intense and suddenly birth seems so imminent. Respond to her fears with the hugest dose of TLC and oodles of reassurance: you can talk her down from that fear-driven self-doubt by reminding her, 'you can do it and you ARE doing it.' If there has ever been a time when a woman needs to hear all the sincere, loving, kind and confidence-inducing words, it is now! Gently remind her just how strong and incredible she really is. This is a very good time to remind her of her favourite affirmations (see page 95) or read her one of her birth letters (see page 148).

- Tension that is building inside her could trigger the fight, flight or freeze response and hold things up, making birth seem more scary, so refer back to her simple primitive needs and be present, see that she is as comfortable as possible, gently encourage her to relax her jaw and make sure that the room is calm, the lights low if possible, and the overall ambience is peaceful.

- At this point she may find touch distracting and irritating. Do not take this personally – it is very normal at this stage. She is likely to be feeling overstimulated sensory-wise, but being strong and present can make all the difference to her and help her feel safe.

- Crack open the frankincense essential oil, known for its soothing effect on heightened emotions. Put one neat drop on the centre of each of her hands, rub it in with your thumbs, then lift her hands up and encourage her to cup them round her nose and mouth and take three slow, deep breaths. The frankincense can also deliver a calming effect on anyone else who is around her at this time as it is inhaled.

- Revisit the grounding and calming acupressure point P6 on (see page 25) to encourage a sense of internal calm and reduce nausea, which can resurface during transition due to the hormonal responses within her birthing body.

Birth Part 3 – A Very Special Delivery

Vaginal birth

During this second stage birthing women will often turn to us and say, through a guttural groan and involuntary push, 'I need a poo!' and that is a really good sign. As the baby starts to move down you are likely to feel the intense sensation of rectal pressure. The temptation here can be to hold your breath as the sensation washes over you, but this is exactly when some releasing downward breathwork (see pages 134–135) can be very powerful. You could also use some lavender essential oil on a cool wet flannel across your forehead or the back of your neck as you will be very warm from all that hard work. Peppermint or orange essential oil on a paper fan can also be an effective pick-me-up to help stimulate and refresh you and give you the zingy boost you may need. Your midwife will work with you and your birth partner to help get you into positions (see opposite and on the following pages) that will encourage a smooth passage for your baby.

Just, how?

It is completely understandable that you may feel concerned and confused as to how in the world your little one will be able to move through this small space and be born. The sums just don't add up, right? However, that's until you understand fully how your baby and your body make a brilliant team and work together for this to happen.

This knowledge is a game changer – your vagina is made to shape-shift. If you pop a clean finger inside of yourself and feel the sides of the vagina, you will notice they are bumpy. That is because the layers of the vaginal walls are gathered up. These pleats of stretchy fibres have already been preparing to expand and unfold with the help of hormones that are present during pregnancy. Once the cervix is fully dilated, the muscular tube of the birth canal stretches and unfolds to accommodate the birth of the baby. What is even more incredible is that once birth is complete and the hormones change with a huge drop in oestrogen and progesterone levels, your vagina uses that elasticity to fold in once again to return to its original shape. Although it might not be exactly as it was pre-kids, the vagina itself does a pretty good job of remodelling itself back to its old shape and size in the six to eight weeks following birth. It really is such an incredibly clever and adaptable organ.

Birth positions

Any position where you are upright, forward and open (UFO) will have gravity working with you, allow your pelvis to open, your tailbone to move more freely and baby will be pushing down on your cervix, which will help you to dilate more effectively!

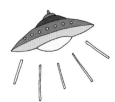

Change positions regularly – moving from one position to the other will help jiggle baby down into the pelvis. Follow your instinct. You will instinctively move to a position that feels right to you.

If in doubt remember UFO – Upright, Forward, Open.

Standing lean

A standing lean is a fab position that allows you to move freely, rest in between surges and ensures gravity is working with you. Standing allows your tailbone to move freely, making space for baby, and is great if you have suffered with hip pain in your pregnancy and early labour.

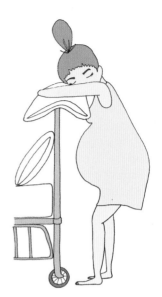

Bed back lean

This wonderful position has all the benefits of the standing lean, but is great if you are feeling a little tired as it allows you to kneel on the bed.

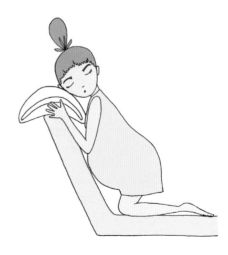

Left lateral side lying

This is fabulous if you are tired and need a rest. Left side lying allows you to relax your body while you labour, which can make contractions more effective. Lying on your left takes the pressure off your main vein – the Vena Cava – ensuring optimum blood flow to the placenta. When it comes to pushing, this position is more powerful if your birth partner holds your leg up for you as this gives you some resistance to push against, while also increasing the opening of the pelvis.

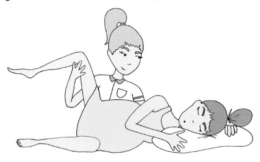

Birthing pool

Being immersed in water can be extremely comforting, and many women find that it lessens the need for pain relief. The buoyancy water provides means that it is very easy to move positions. It also softens the muscles of the perineum which increases their elasticity and can help prevent tearing. The birthing pool has the added benefit of feeling like a private space for women, making you feel less observed, which can help to reduce anxiety and inhibitions.

The final push

Your birth team will be by your side to encourage you through the final pushes so that you can finally meet your baby. As the head edges further forwards, bit by bit you are likely to feel a strong stretching that may present itself as a stinging or burning sensation. Often women respond by actively pushing the baby down hard, but if everything is progressing as expected you can let those involuntary pushes do the work and keep on focusing on your breath.

Assisted delivery

Occasionally, if mum is completely exhausted or if her baby is showing some signs of distress, it may be that some help is needed in these final stages. An assisted delivery will involve a doctor using either a ventouse (suction cup) or forceps (a delivery instrument that looks like metal salad tongs) to help bring your baby down and result in birth.

If you experience an assisted delivery at the end of your labour, make sure you and your birth partner fully understand why this pathway has been taken for you and your baby, so that you really feel like you are a part of the decision-making process.

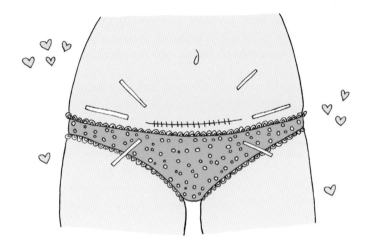

Abdominal birth

Birth is unpredictable and sometimes the decision has to be made to perform a surgical procedure – a caesarean section – to keep mum and baby safe. During this procedure your baby will be delivered in theatre, through incisions in the abdomen and uterus. Whether you have chosen to have a C-section, have been advised to book one because you are carrying more than one baby, or for other medical reasons, or maybe birth suddenly takes a turn down the surgical path, below are our top tips for having a gentle and positive abdominal birth.

- Have a calming meditation track or some calming music to listen to while you are waiting to go into theatre.

- You can ask for the fabric screen to be lowered so that you can see your beautiful baby being born (don't worry, you won't be able to see the opening).

- If you and baby are well, you can ask for the cord clamping to be a little delayed, to ensure your baby gets the nutrient-rich blood from the placenta.

- You can have skin-to-skin time with your baby, and if baby is well, they can remain with you while you are being sutured.

- You can ask for your own music to be played in the room.

- If you don't know what sex you are having you can ask that your partner announce that to you once baby is born.

- You can ask your birth team to lower the lighting on your side of the screen so that it isn't too bright for baby while you are having your lovely skin-to-skin.

Your recovery after a C-section
Your midwife will give you hospital painkillers while you are there. Take them regularly to keep yourself as comfortable as possible. And do press the buzzer and call for help whenever you need it! Remember, you are recovering from surgery, so it's important to rest and accept all the help.

Once you are home, continue to rest. You will need someone to look after you as you as you shouldn't be lifting anything heavier than your baby!

TOP TIPS FOR YOUR COMFORT

- Buy big, cotton high-waisted pants that won't sit on the scar. They will also hold you in, which will feel comforting.

- Remember you will still bleed after a C-section so don't forget maternity pads.

- Have lots of pillows readily available to prop you up, lay baby on during a feed so that they are not resting on your tummy, and to hug while you cough or laugh, to support your scar.

- Use a hot water bottle to warm your ribs and upper back where you can experience trapped wind post-surgery (note: do not use the hot water bottle on your abdomen / scar area).

- Stock up on painkillers and peppermint tea, which is great to help relieve the pain caused by trapped wind.

- Sometimes it can take a little longer for the milk to come in after an abdominal birth so if you are planning to breastfeed, keep having lots of skin-to-skin contact and keep putting baby to the breast to help bring the milk in. Harvesting colostrum a few days before your section can also help (see pages 156–157).

DOES THIS MEAN I WILL HAVE TO HAVE ANOTHER C-SECTION NEXT TIME?

Having an abdominal birth this time doesn't always mean you will have to have one next time. Some women choose to have another C-section, but if you and baby are well and the pregnancy is uncomplicated then many women go on to have a VBAC (Vaginal Birth After Caesarean) with their next birth.

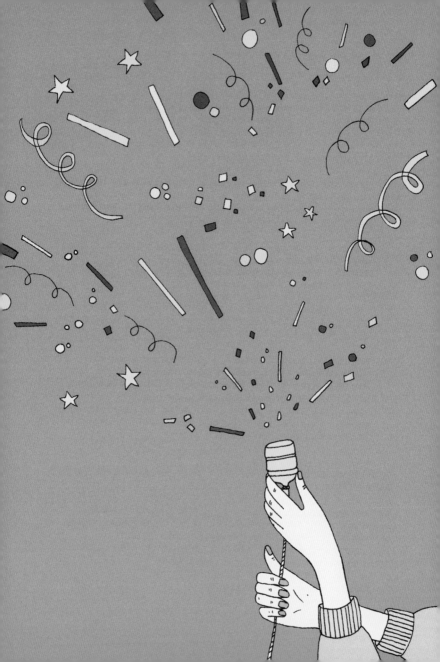

You Did It!

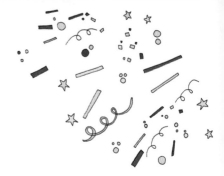

You. Did. It!! And after all these months your baby is finally here! You may be overcome with emotion and relief and not know whether to laugh or cry – so maybe you do a bit of both. You may also feel sudden complete exhaustion, as if all the energy has been sucked right out of you. You might experience an oxytocin high, or just shock as adrenaline takes over and you tremble and shake while your body tries to reset itself.

Each one of these responses is completely normal. You have just birthed your baby. In a way, this moment can sometimes feel too big to get your head around initially. You have made an actual human and they are here with you at last, after having journeyed through one the most physical and psychological rollercoasters of your life. Like a marathon runner making it past the finish line, it's an incredible moment that truly feels outside of time and space.

Unless there is a reason to take baby away to be checked, your little one will be placed on you for some skin-to-skin time. This is very beneficial to them (as you will see in the next section) but it's also a really good way to help you take your time to take it all in, slowly and calmly, as your body digests the news that the baby has been born and sends hormones to your uterus to release the placenta. Don't worry, remember the placenta is soft and malleable and you won't need to put much effort into pushing it out. Your midwife will guide you through the whole process.

If your placenta is taking its sweet time to release, your midwife will be keeping a close eye on you, but do try the following ways to help nature along:

- Hydrate – have some water or coconut water.
- Have something sugary, like a few jelly babies. If you can't face food, some sips of sugary tea or a spoonful of date syrup or honey will do the job.
- Stay warm – this stops the muscles from contracting and will keep tissues soft.
- Have lots of skin-to-skin with your baby where possible and try to latch them for a feed. Nipple stimulation is great for placenta release.
- Sit on the loo! This can open the pelvis and is a good position to birth your placenta.

Your midwife will gently check you and the baby, and if they are happy that you both seem well then it is likely they will take a step back and just let you have some blissful moments together.

Don't worry

Some women say to us that when they saw their baby, they thought they were sweet little things, but didn't feel a rush of immediate love – and that worried them. You would be surprised how common this can be. Sometimes it's only days or even weeks later, in your home environment, adjusting to your new life with your baby, that the love starts to grow. However, if you're concerned as the weeks go on you can always mention it to your GP or health visitor, but know that there is no timeframe here and the huge rise and fall of hormones can play a significant part in the bonding process.

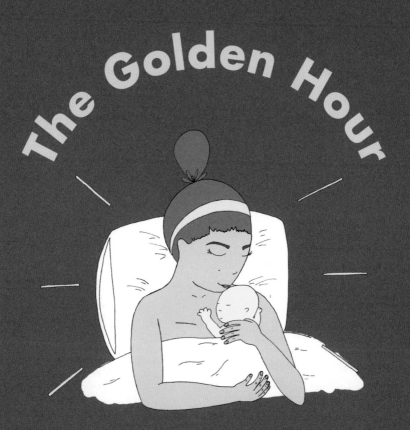

The Golden Hour

The golden hour refers to that magical time immediately after your baby has been born and placed on you, where you get to unwrap them from their cosy blankets like the best present you've ever had and finally meet the little human that YOU grew!

During this time, it is widely encouraged for you to spend an uninterrupted hour of skin-to-skin with your brand new little one. Providing all is okay, your midwife is likely to make sure you and your baby are comfortable, check your blood loss is

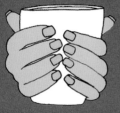

within normal limits and will then take a step back busying herself with writing up her notes and going to get you a sweet tea and toast to give you a little energy boost.

Keep your golden hour environment as calm and tranquil as possible. Continue with low lighting, gentle music or quiet conversations and take in those precious newborn moments.

Benefits for you

- Encourages oxytocin release which can support bonding, contract your uterus down (therefore helping to prevent heavy bleeding) and encourage the release of colostrum if you are breastfeeding.

- Helps lower your cortisol levels (stress hormone) and decrease feeling physically and mentally shocked following birth.

- Calms and regulates your breathing and heartbeat which may feel like they are racing after birth.

- Gives you an opportunity to see, touch, smell, hear and hold your baby undisturbed.

Benefits for baby

- Keeps the baby warm immediately after birth as the evaporation of the amniotic fluid on their skin can cool them down quickly. You are like a radiator to them and they will be warm and contained in between you and the towels/blankets.

- Encourages them to release oxytocin and down-regulate their high cortisol levels after being born.

- Provides comfort and familiarity through hearing your voice, recognising your smell, feeling the rhythm of your breathing and heartbeat. This helps to regulate their heartbeat as they lie against you.

Recreating the Golden Hour

Occasionally, there may be medical reasons that prevent you and your baby from having a full hour together following birth, but remember, skin-to-skin is a beautiful way to soothe, regulate and comfort yourself and your baby throughout the weeks and months ahead, not just immediately after birthing.

To encourage oxytocin to flow, find a gently lit, quiet space and place your baby on the centre of your chest. This could be sitting up on the sofa or upright in bed with a blanket around you both or having a warming bath together. Doing this regularly can promote bonding and connection and can be used when breast- or bottle-feeding your little one.

FIRST 24 HOURS CRIB SHEET

Once baby is born, your birth team will continue to look after you both. Remember, birthing your baby is incredible and intense and you may be feeling all the feels right now so do ask for help and support any time you need it. It can be helpful to know roughly what the next 24 hours will look like - so here's a little breakdown of what happens next. The order of events may vary depending on your birth.

GOLDEN HOUR

- Skin-to-skin to regulate baby's temperature, breathing and heartbeat, plus precious time to get a good look at your baby for the first time.

- Baby's first feed.

- Delayed cord clamping where possible to enable the cord to run clear so that baby gets all the lovely blood supply meant for them.

- Suturing or 'closing' if in theatre following a C-section. Transferred round to recovery area after surgery is complete.

- Delivery of the placenta / blood pressure check / observations of blood loss.

- Time to be left alone to bond with baby.

- Tea and toast, or your post-birth picnic — you will probably feel VERY hungry!

HOUR TWO

- Stitches (if required. This may need to be done earlier if there are concerns with bleeding.)

- Baby checked from top to toe, weighed, measured, vitamin k given.

- Birth partner, mum or midwife to dress baby for the first time (depending on your wishes).

- More precious cuddles from parents and dazzled staring at the baby.

HOUR THREE ONWARDS

- Baby will likely be exhausted from birth and will nod off to sleep.

- You will probably be transferred to a bed on the postnatal ward.

- You may wish to have a shower and get into some fresh, cosy clothes.

- Although you may feel wide awake with adrenaline and obsessed by your beautiful baby, try to sleep or at least rest as you will need your energy again later when baby gets hungry.

- More checks with the midwife for blood loss, blood pressure and temperature.

HOURS SIX TO SEVEN

- Baby may wake around now feeling a bit hungry and benefiting from some skin-to-skin as they continue their transition into life outside the womb.

- You may be discharged home if it is a day-time hour and you and the baby have no risk factors. This will be delayed until the morning if you birth late in the day or during the night, have any health issues that they want to keep a closer eye on, or need more support with infant feeding.

Note: If you remain in hospital over the next 24 hours you will usually be having blood pressure/blood loss observations and infant feeding support from your midwife every 4—6 hours.

AT HOME

- When you get home, change into your comfiest, softest, cosiest clothes, get your partner to pop the kettle on and have a few moments just to take it all in — you are at home with your brand-new baby!

- Continue with plenty of skin-to-skin.

- Have minimal visitors as you and your partner are likely to be exhausted.

- Carry on with 3—4 hourly feeds, depending on what your midwife told you.

- Call the hospital up and speak with a community midwife if you have ANY worries or questions.

- Your midwife team will continue to check on you for the next 5—10 days, and you will have a number to call if you have any worries or concerns.

- Your focus now should be on resting, feeding and getting to know your baby. Accept all offers of help and don't be afraid to ask for more if you need it. You will need a little time to recover from birth and soon you'll be feeling strong again, but right now you need to give your body a huge dose of TLC.

a final word . . .

As the Superwomen we are, we give so much of ourselves up to growing our little bean during pregnancy. Perhaps we are also looking after other children, and the days and nights can be busy and sleep deprived. We want you to remember just how important you are, too. Your wellbeing matters because you need to be fit and strong to care for your baby when it arrives, and you can only do this if you look after yourself.

What we know about caring for ourselves and keeping on top of aches and pains and mental fatigue is that it's the little things that count. A bath, a foot rub, an early night. It's all those little moments of self-care spread over the week that will have way more benefit than a day off to go to the spa or shops once or twice a year!

Don't get us wrong, those bigger treats are lovely too, but don't hold out for 'once in a blue moon' moments – schedule in self-care daily. It doesn't have to be anything grand, just regular little acts of kindness aimed at yourself instead of everyone else. Come on, look at what your body is doing right now; you really are worth it!

Keep this book handy so that you can turn to it any time you need a bit of self-care advice, a little tip or trick along the way, or maybe some TLC and reassurance. It's all in here, and it all comes from a place of understanding the highs and lows that come with pregnancy and birth from our experience of supporting women on this epic journey.

If you have a partner, or a friend or family member who plans to help you through pregnancy and the birth, make sure they have a good read through the book too so that they can understand how best to support you.

It is so important to keep that self-care going into the postnatal period. All too often we've seen women completely forget their own wellbeing in those early weeks as they juggle life with a newborn and all the demands this brings. We know it's a rollercoaster, but we also know that we can ride that rollercoaster with way less impact on our mental and physical wellbeing if we look after ourselves as well as we look after the little ones.

We've had the absolute privilege to train in cultures where women are encouraged to rest for 40 days after the birth of their baby, where all responsibilities other than feeding her baby and resting are taken away, and where she is massaged and fed nourishing foods until she is fully recovered from the birth. We know our society isn't set up in a way that makes it easy for us to replicate that level of care, however we do know that we can achieve something a little similar.

We want to take this final moment to remind you that you are awesome, you will be an amazing mother, or mother to more than one, and wish you heaps of happiness on this adventure of a lifetime.

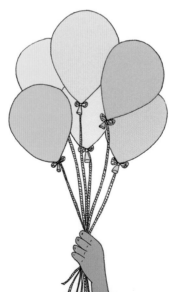

Index:

Resources

Perinatal mental health
www.bestbeginnings.org.uk
www.mentalhealth.org.uk
www.mind.org.uk
www.nhs.uk
www.pandasfoundation.org.uk
www.pregnancysicknesssupport.org.uk
www.samaritans.org–08457909090 (24hrs)

Baby positioning
www.spinningbabies.com
www.tommys.org

General
www.babcycentre.co.uk
www.sarawickham.com
www.tommys.org

Antenatal Education
www.birthrights.org.uk
www.bumpandbabyclub.com
www.childbirthconnection.org
www.pelvicpartnership.org.uk

Wellbeing
www.beccyhands.co.uk
www.brightonphysio.co.uk
www.headspace.com
www.kiranjot.com
www.mindfulmotherhood.org
www.pregnancysicknesssupport.org.uk

General help and support
www.doula.org.uk

Thank you! ♥

First and foremost, thank you to our brilliant publisher Sam Jackson (and all at Penguin) who put her faith in us once again, because she understands how empowering it is to feel supported and well informed.

Thank you to our very talented editor Laura Herring and her eagle eyes; once again we won the editor lottery with you!

Next a big thank you to our wonderfully creative designers Laura Liggins, and Nikki Dupin at Studio nic&lou who turned a monochrome manuscript into the stylish little hardback you see today.

Thank you to our dear friend and illustrator Kay Train who we have had the pleasure of working with again on this amazing new project. Kay, we love you! You have the ability to bring our words to life, and your illustrations give us all the feels.

Thank you to Tina Mason and Kiranjot for all the amazing work you do with women and for contributing to this book with your expertise, and thank you to all the mums who shared their stories with us that are scattered throughout this book.

Alexis would also like to thank: Jean, Mimi, Amy, Denise and Gemma, who have taught me most of what I know about being a midwife. Thanks to my mum and little sister for your never-ending support. My dad for all the love and encouragement you ever gave me, that I still feel even though you are no longer here. And to my brilliant husband Dan who has had my back and believed in everything I have ever done since we met back at school, 20 years ago. And thank you to my three lovely littles who are super-proud of the books we've written and wondered if they could dress up as me for World Book Day.

Beccy would like to thank: all of the amazing teachers I have trained and worked with through the years. Learning from you all, with your very different approaches to pregnancy and birth support, has given me an amazingly nurturing and varied outlook in my work. Thanks to my family and friends for your constant support. Thank you to my amazing husband Barney for always believing in me, and always making me see the positives. And finally, thanks to my two wonderful daughters: having you will always be the best thing I have ever done! Life, although loud and busy, is so much better with you both in it!

Finally, we'd like to say a huge thank you to all of the women we have worked with throughout our professional careers. We learn so much from you all, and it is an absolute honour, always. If it wasn't for all of you, we wouldn't be here doing what we are doing today.